Hospital Pre-registration Pharmacist Training

TOMORROW'S PHARMACIST

Welcome to *Tomorrow's Pharmacist* series – helping you with your future career in pharmacy.

Like the journal, book titles under this banner are specifically aimed at pre-registration trainees and pharmacy students to help them prepare for their future career. These books provide guidance on topics such as the interview and application process for the pre-registration year, the registration examination and future employment in a specific specialty.

The annual journal *Tomorrow's Pharmacist* will contain information and excerpts from the books in this series.

You can find more information on the journal at www.pjonline.com/tp

Titles in the series so far include:
The Pre-registration Interview: Preparation for the application process
Registration Exam Questions
MCQs in Pharmaceutical Calculations
Hospital Pre-registration Pharmacist Training

Hospital Pre-registration Pharmacist Training

Aamer Safdar

BPharm, MSc, PGCE, MA, MRPharmS, FHEA

Principal Pharmacist Lead for Education and Development,
Guy's and St Thomas' NHS Foundation Trust, London
RPSGB Pre-registration Tutor and Manager

and

Shirley Ip

BPharm, MRPharmS, PGCE

Lead Pharmacist – Care of Older People, Whittington NHS Trust,
London
RPSGB Pre-registration Tutor

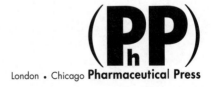

London • Chicago **Pharmaceutical Press**

Published by the Pharmaceutical Press
An imprint of RPS Publishing

1 Lambeth High Street, London SE1 7JN, UK
100 South Atkinson Road, Suite 200, Grayslake, IL 60030-7820, USA

© Pharmaceutical Press 2009

(**PP**) is a trade mark of RPS Publishing
RPS Publishing is the publishing organisation of the Royal Pharmaceutical Society
of Great Britain

First published 2009

Typeset by Thomson Digital (India) Limited, Noida
Printed in Great Britain by TJ International Ltd, Padstow, Cornwall

ISBN 978 0 85369 785 5

Contents

Preface

From our involvement with pre-registration training for almost all of our careers in different guises, and more recently the management of the pre-registration programme at Guy's and St Thomas' NHS Foundation Trust, we thought that it would be useful to put our experiences into a book for others to share and benefit from. The idea originated when Aamer was in charge of the pre-registration programme and his trainees often said to him 'You have so many stories, you could write a book'; well after a number of years this is indeed what we have done.

We hope that this book will benefit those of you who are either considering hospital pharmacy as your chosen area for pre-registration training or currently in a hospital pre-registration placement. We hope that by reading our book you realise that you are not the only ones having these training experiences; this is particularly the case for those of you who are in smaller pre-registration teams when there is no one else to talk to and share your experiences – good or bad.

Although the book is focused primarily on hospital pharmacy, we anticipate that many of the things that we discuss are equally applicable in any other sector of pharmacy.

We hope that you enjoy reading our book because this is the first book of its type focusing on the actual experiences, and emotions, of completing a hospital pre-registration training year.

Aamer Safdar and Shirley Ip
May, 2009

Acknowledgements

We would like to dedicate this book to all our pre-regs who in their own way have contributed greatly to its content, especially some of the more unusual anecdotes and experiences. We are not going to name names, but you will know who you are when you read what you said or did while you were pre-regs under our care!

Although we have invested much time, energy, sweat and sometimes blood in supporting and training pre-regs, they are only with us for 1 year and the fact that many of them have gone on to take up responsible positions in the pharmacy profession is a testament to the pre-regs themselves.

The reason for writing this book is simply for pre-regs because they don't always get the support that they sometimes need and don't always want to raise their inner worries and concerns.

It would be remiss of us not to acknowledge the members of the pharmacy departments with which we have worked who have been invaluable in supporting pre-reg trainees in all respects. Without this support our jobs as pre-reg trainers and then tutors would be impossible.

About the authors

Aamer graduated from the School of Pharmacy and completed his pre-registration year at Guy's and St Thomas' NHS Foundation Trust. Aamer then stayed at Guy's and St Thomas' for most of his career in a variety of posts, starting with resident pharmacist; he left the Trust to work at the then Lambeth, Southwark and Lewisham Health Authority as a prescribing adviser for a short while. He returned to Guy's and St Thomas' as Specialist Pharmacist in Oncology, before moving to a dispensary/clinical role, where he was first introduced to pre-registration training as he took an interest in training and assessing pre-registration trainees.

Aamer then decided that it was time for a change and left the Trust to undertake a 1-year full-time MSc course in Clinical Pharmacy at the School of Pharmacy. He undertook a variety of locum positions in hospital pharmacy before starting the course. After completing his MSc, Aamer returned to Guy's and St Thomas' in the position of pre-registration pharmacist facilitator. While in this post Aamer completed a postgraduate certificate in education at the University of Greenwich. Following an internal promotion and then re-grading in line with the Agenda for Change, Aamer took on more teaching responsibilities.

Aamer completed a Master of Arts in Management Studies at the University of Greenwich and became a Fellow of the Higher Education Academy. He is involved with teaching and tutoring students at postgraduate level and with courses at Diploma and Masters levels, including the MSc in Clinical Pharmacy International Practice and Policy for international pharmacists.

Aamer's current position is Principal Pharmacist Lead for Education and Development where he has a wide range of educational and managerial responsibilities.

Shirley graduated from the School of Pharmacy and completed her pre-registration year at the Royal Surrey County Hospital in Guildford. She then worked at Greenwich District General Hospital in London until the hospital closed and all services moved to the Queen Elizabeth Hospital, in nearby

Woolwich, south-east London. Shirley undertook a variety of roles at the Queen Elizabeth Hospital including Medicines Management Project Pharmacist (setting up one-stop dispensing in the hospital), Medicines Management and Formulary Pharmacist, and finally Education and Training Pharmacist, while providing a pharmaceutical service to a number of different wards and specialities.

Shirley was first introduced to pre-registration training when she was asked to supervise pre-regs during their clinical rotations, and eventually became involved with clinical training and mentoring of both pre-regs and junior pharmacists, including intensive remedial work with staff who needed extra input to improve their performance.

Shirley joined Guy's and St Thomas' as Senior Pharmacist for Education and Development to concentrate her efforts on development of her training skills. She was involved with the coordination and management of pre-registration training and the teaching and assessment of pre-registration pharmacists. While in this role Shirley completed a postgraduate certificate in education at the University of Greenwich. Shirley's post was shared across Guy's and St Thomas' NHS Foundation Trust and Southwark Primary Care Trust where she has been involved with the development of an innovative hospital/PCT split pre-reg programme, together with increasing exposure of pre-registration trainees to PCT and other sectors of pharmacy such as prison pharmacy.

Shirley is currently working at the Whittington Hospital as the Lead Pharmacist for Care of Older People and remains involved with training pre-registration pharmacists, pharmacy and medical undergraduates and supporting newly qualified pharmacists.

Introduction

'A wise man learns from experience, an even wiser man learns from the experience of others ...' Plato (424–423 to 348–347 BC).

The pre-registration year is one of the most challenging years of your career. Every pharmacist has to undergo this year and can probably remember something that he or she learned from the pre-registration year, in some cases at a push!

The Royal Pharmaceutical Society of Great Britain (RPSGB) defines the training required and sets out a set of performance standards and an examination syllabus for the registration exam. Many pre-registration trainees see the registration exam as the most important aspect of the pre-registration year, whereas many tutors see the competency-based training aspect as the most important.

At this stage it is important to mention some of the statutory requirements of the pre-registration year, although this book does not focus on this. Up-to-date information about the year can be obtained from the RPSGB website: www.rpsgb.org. There are other textbooks that discuss some of the requirements about pre-registration training such as the *Pharmacy Pre-registration Handbook* by Lindsay M Taylor, published by Pharmaceutical Press.

Pre-registration training is the period of employment that pharmacy graduates must successfully complete before they can register as pharmacists in the UK. In most cases this is a 1-year training period immediately after the pharmacy degree; for sandwich course students it is integrated with their undergraduate studies.

The pre-registration training year consists of 52 weeks of satisfactory supervised and assessed training in employment. Each trainee must then pass the registration examination for admission to the register. Each trainee has a designated pre-registration tutor within the employing organisation who formally assesses the trainee every 13 weeks. Trainees are eligible to sit the registration examination after a satisfactory 39-week progress report and after completing 45 weeks of training. There is a final assessment at 50 weeks and a final declaration by the tutor. Once the registration examination has been passed and the 52 weeks of satisfactory training have been completed and the other requirements met (such as providing a health declaration), applicants can be entered on the register. Entry on the register confers the award of Member of the Royal Pharmaceutical Society (MRPharmS).

This work-based training is in an RPSGB-accredited training premises which can be a hospital, community pharmacy, pharmaceutical industry or even a primary care trust (PCT). Depending on the programme that you are following, there may be an opportunity for you to spend 2–4 weeks in the community pharmacy sector; this experience is not mandatory and not all hospitals offer it. A full list of current accredited training places can be found on the RPSGB website.

As a pre-registration trainee, you need to complete this training and be assessed against the 76 performance standards by your tutor before being signed off as 'competent' at the end of the year, as well as passing the registration exam. This book concentrates on this aspect of the training year and provides some of our thoughts and experiences of how to succeed and get through the year.

We start the book at the point of starting the training year, rather than how to get into hospital pharmacy for your pre-registration year. Nadia Bukhari's book *The Pre-registration Interview* (Pharmaceutical Press) already covers this, and there may some aspects that we also cover, such as what an employer looks for, but we recommend that prospective students have a look at Nadia's book for advice and tips about the interview process.

As the book starts at the beginning of the year we have gone through a typical hospital pharmacy pre-registration programme, although we recognise that locally each hospital trust has its own way of doing things and offers different rotations and experiences. We have based the content of the book on our joint experiences of working in a large London teaching hospital and in a local district general hospital where the role of the pre-registration trainee can be very different. With this in mind, we have not covered everything that you will experience in your year and indeed there may be things that we discuss that are not covered in your year at all.

We have gone through the initial few weeks of working, which include getting to know your fellow trainees and your tutor, as well as the workplace in which you are going to spend the next 12 months. The next section of the book provides some detail about each rotation that you do. Most hospitals offer very similar rotations although the experiences, roles and responsibilities of trainees are different depending on the type of hospital pharmacy that you are in. We provide hints and tips of how to succeed throughout and summarise these at the end of each section.

Where possible, we have supported our comments by using direct quotes from previous pre-reg trainees. As part of our ongoing quality assurance of our pre-reg year, we captured and recorded quotes from our pre-regs and have used these in this book. For obvious reasons we have kept the details of the pre-regs anonymous.

There is inevitably a section on preparing for, and getting through, the registration exam but we do not focus on the content of the exam and what to revise because there are other books for this; we have shared our experiences of what to do and what not to do. There is some duplication with other books and we recommend that, if you would like further advice about the registration exam, you take a look at these books as well as at the RPSGB website.

There is a section on preparing for the next stages of your career and we share some thoughts of our trainees who have gone on to make their first steps as pharmacists.

We finish with a section on some specialist programmes and how they can be managed; these are mainly split 6-month placements where the emphasis on the performance standards is much higher than in a 12-month programme.

At the time of writing, we recognise that the face of pharmacy education is changing radically and in a few years' time pre-registration training will look significantly different to how it looks now. The introduction of an integrated pharmacy degree programme will change how training is delivered and how assessment is carried out, but we believe that many of the experiences in this book will hold irrespective of how and where the training is undertaken.

It is important to note that the RPSGB will no longer exist in its current form after 2010 and all regulatory functions will be the responsibility of the General Pharmaceutical Council (GPhC). These will include regulation of pharmacy education and pre-registration training. At the time of writing, the RPSGB regulates pre-registration training and all references to the RPSGB should be superseded by the GPhC after 2010.

Before we start the book, there are some important terms that you may need to become familiar with!

Once you start the pre-registration year, initially you are known as 'a pre-reg', or perhaps 'the pre-reg', or if you are in a team then 'the pre-regs'. The official title for your post is also varied: pre-registration pharmacist, pre-registration pharmacist trainee, pre-registration graduate or pre-registration student! The terms applied to the training year are also different; the year is generally known as 'the pre-reg' or 'the pre-reg year'. From now on we refer to the pre-registration year as 'the pre-reg year' and you are known as 'the pre-regs'. Interestingly, or perhaps not so interestingly, there is no consensus on whether it is pre-registration or preregistration – there have been many arguments over the use of the hyphen! Throughout this book, we use the term 'pre-regs'.

REFERENCES

Bukhari N. *The Pre-registration Interview: Preparation for the application process*. London: Pharmaceutical Press, 2007.

Taylor LM. *Pharmacy Pre-registration Handbook*. London: Pharmaceutical Press, 2002.

Section 1

Pre-registration trainees

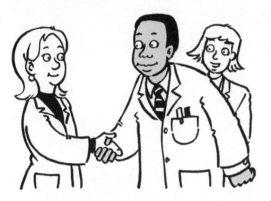

Expectations of the pre-registration placement

Congratulations! You've just got yourself a Masters degree and had the graduation ceremony and have got yourself a job as a 'pre-registration pharmacist'. You're on top of the world! You've seen it all and done it all during your 4 years at university and you can't wait to start your pre-reg placement to put into practice everything that you've learned.

Be careful though! We're warning you now that, when you start your pre-reg placement, you will NOT be treated as a 'pharmacist' even though 'pre-registration pharmacist' is your job title. You will also not *feel* like a pharmacist. The position that you hold is definitely a trainee position, and you are there to learn, on top of delivering some aspect of the pharmacy service. You will feel like you have come from the top of the pile and landed firmly at the bottom once again. And you will probably get that feeling every time that you start a new rotation and learn a new skill.

Another word of warning is that, although you are a 'pre-registration pharmacist', you are not legally allowed to call yourself a 'pharmacist' until you are registered with the Royal Pharmaceutical Society of Great Britain (RPSGB) as a registered, practising pharmacist, and that happens only when you have fulfilled all of the RPSGB performance standards and passed the registration examination, and your pre-reg tutor has signed you off as being fit to be a pharmacist. So, do NOT introduce yourself as a pharmacist to patients or other healthcare professionals, because you can't call yourself that – yet.

You need to think about how you are going to introduce yourself to patients and other healthcare staff. It is worth noting that pre-reg house officers (PRHOs) are qualified doctors in their first years of foundation training, and are known as FY1s or FY2s, whereas a pre-reg pharmacist has not yet qualified as a pharmacist. Some pre-regs call themselves students or trainees whereas others say that they are 'from pharmacy'. You will need to find out from your workplace what their preference for you is because to call yourself a pharmacist when you are not is illegal.

When you start work, expectations from the staff will vary wildly. This may be slightly confusing. What standing you have in your pharmacy as a 'pre-reg' depends entirely on the culture of your workplace, and more specifically on the views that the people with whom you work have with regard to 'pre-regs'. It also depends on what jobs a pre-reg is supposed to do at your workplace. In some hospitals you will be given a lot of responsibility and chucked in at the deep end right from the start, but in others your level of responsibility will grow as you progress throughout the training year. In addition, some people 'like' pre-regs and understand the whole point of pre-reg training, but many others do not!

The confusion is understandable because, although you are not students anymore, you are certainly not independent practitioners yet; you still need a lot of training (especially at the beginning of the year) to enable you to do anything at all and, by the end of the training year, you are expected to be a fully functioning pharmacist and may well be in charge of the people who have given you training throughout your pre-reg year.

> 'In terms of making decisions I feel very protected because I'm not allowed to do anything without supervision. Having come from a community background where I used to act with some autonomy, I'm finding this supervision smothering already.'

The first thing to say about your pre-reg placement is that you are a salaried employee, and therefore you are being paid to work. Becoming an actual employee may come as a bit of a shock to many of you, but this change in your status means that there needs to be a corresponding change of attitude.

As a student, did you find it hard to get out of bed and turn up to your 9 am lectures? Did you decide where and which classes you attended? Did you somehow accidentally end up having 3-hour lunch breaks? Did you work half-heartedly at some of the subjects that you weren't so interested in? Were you always late, if you ever showed up at all?

Of course you did – you were a student! Needless to say, this type of behaviour would be frowned upon in a workplace.

When you start work you need to bear in mind some really simple things that people who have had some experience of (having worked before) might take for granted.

As you will be working in a workplace, so you will be working with professionals and so you need to turn up to work on time and look professional (no more uni days). You will be working with many different types of professionals within the workplace and also with many different types of people as patients, so you need to present a 'professional' persona while in the workplace.

So, what do we mean exactly when we say 'professional'? If you look at a dictionary the definition is something like the following (from http:// dictionary.reference.com):

1. Following an occupation as a means of livelihood or for gain: a *professional builder.*
2. Of, pertaining to, or connected with a profession: *professional studies.*
3. Appropriate to a profession: *professional objectivity.*
4. Engaged in one of the learned professions: *a lawyer is a professional person.*
5. Following as a business an occupation ordinarily engaged in as a pastime: *a professional golfer.*
6. Making a business or constant practice of something not properly to be regarded as a business: 'A salesman,' he said, 'is a professional optimist.'
7. Undertaken or engaged in as a means of livelihood or for gain: *professional baseball.*
8. Of or for a professional person or his or her place of business or work: *a professional apartment; professional equipment.*
9. Done by a professional; expert: *professional car repairs.*

Being a professional is defined as the following (from http://dictionary. reference.com):

- A person who belongs to one of the professions, especially one of the learned professions.
- A person who earns a living in a sport or other occupation frequently engaged in by amateurs: *golf professional.*
- An expert player, as of golf or tennis, serving as a teacher, consultant, performer or contestant: *pro.*
- A person who is expert at his or her work: *you can tell by her comments that this editor is a real professional.*

A more academic example of professionalism is:

'Professionalism is demonstrated through a foundation of clinical competence, communication skills, and ethical and legal understanding upon which is built the aspiration to and wise application of the principles of professionalism, excellence, humanism, accountability & altruism.' (Stern, 2006, page 19)

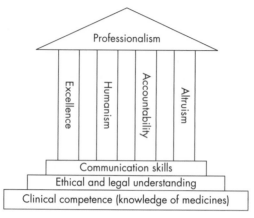

Figure 1.1 A definition of professionalism. (Reproduced with permission from Stern, 2006.)

In professionalism:

- excellence is a commitment to competence and a desire to exceed ordinary standards
- accountability includes self-regulation, standard setting, managing conflicts of interest and the acceptance of responsibility
- altruism is ensuring that pharmacists act in the best interests of patients and not self-interest
- humanism is behaving with respect, compassion, empathy, honour and integrity.

We actually don't mean any of the above when we say that you need to be 'professional'! Being professional (to us) means that you need to display a set of behaviours that would normally be acceptable for somebody who has the same standing, and in the same environment as you, providing a particular service. So, what do you need to do to be professional? We think that there are many different facets, including the following:

- Timekeeping: being on time is very important and completing work to deadlines is also very important. When you are in your rotations, you are expected to do many things at the same time, so organising and prioritising your work to enable you to deliver all your work to the required deadlines are important.
- Dressing appropriately: different workplaces have different dress codes, so the key word here is 'appropriately'. You need to measure yourself by what is deemed acceptable in the workplace that you are in.

Whatever the dress code is, try to create a professional image. Make sure that you wear clean and appropriate clothing, and pay attention to grooming and personal cleanliness. How would it make you feel if you went to a hospital and were confronted by staff who were not very clean? It would make you think that the hospital was not clean, which brings on the fact that you will be seen by patients as a representative of your organisation and not necessarily as an individual. This is something to bear in mind when you present yourself to the outside world.

- Another issue working in healthcare is knowing what you are talking about. At university, if you do not know something you can bluff your way through and hope that you can pick up some points in an exam somewhere along the way; in a work situation, probably involving patients' wellbeing, you had better be sure that you check your facts otherwise harm may come to them and that is not acceptable.

- Completing work to deadlines is a very important skill to develop too – at university maybe your final mark might have suffered due to the late handing in of work; in a work environment, once again, finding the right answer in time may prevent harm to your patient.

- Having an approachable and helpful persona helps you to fit into the work team.

- Being respectful to other people without being a pushover is also a very useful (but hard) skill to have. You need to present yourself in a business-like manner, whether you interact with people in person, on the phone, via email or by writing.

- Also, no matter whether or not you did well in your degree, the test of a professional is how all that knowledge is applied in the workplace, which means that you need to show some common sense. No one said that being professional was going to be easy!

As part of your employment contract you will have an allocated number of days that you can take off as annual leave; the current number of days is 27 and, in some organisations, is split pro rata into the NHS year (April to March), meaning that you need to have taken a number of days by the end of March of your year, with the rest being carried forward into the remainder of your year.

During your university days, there would have been regular breaks at the start/end and mid-semester – half-term holidays do not feature! This means that you should try to spread your annual leave evenly throughout the year; in some rotations they may require you to take a certain proportion of your allowance to ensure that you do not take lots of annual leave in one block, leaving a particular rotation without a pre-reg for a long time. As you will probably be the newest member of staff, and one of the most junior, you will have very little time in which to think about, and apply for, annual leave hotspots such as the Christmas/New Year period; unless you can get in quick enough and plead your case, you may find yourself working some of this time.

Please be aware that the RPSGB states that you need to have completed a certain number of weeks of training by the time that you take your exam. This means that if you have had any extended period of sickness you will need to check whether or not you are eligible to sit the registration exam under the RPSGB byelaws; more information can be obtained from your pre-reg tutor or manager. If you have been sick for an extended period of time, you may be asked to extend your pre-reg training period to comply with the minimum number of weeks or you may need to forfeit some of your annual leave allocation. This is at the discretion of your pre-reg tutor who will seek guidance from both the RPSGB and the human resources team at the hospital.

Also, remember that, unlike university where you chose to be in classes when you wanted to, as an employee you are required to turn up to work unless you have notified your relevant managers otherwise. Any unauthorised absence from work will probably be dealt with severely in a formal manner. There are health and safety issues surrounding everybody knowing where you are.

Wherever you are doing your pre-reg placement you will have a range of different learning experiences offered to you. These 'learning experiences' are normally presented as a number of different rotations in different areas of the pharmacy. While at university, you were told what to learn and how to learn it. During your pre-reg placement, the situation is very different. You will be treated as an adult and need to take responsibility for your own learning.

While you work through your various rotations, it can be very easy to blindly do what people tell you to do without thinking about things. It is up to you to make the most of your pre-reg year. The motivation for your success in this year should come from within.

The flipside to this is that you mustn't try to run before you can walk. Remember that you must learn the mundane and routine things first, so that you have a good grounding of how things work (such as how medicines are procured, stored and distributed to the wards), before you move on to learning the more complicated, 'sexy', clinical things. Remember that everything that you learn during your pre-reg year is important, even though you may not know the relevance of what you are doing at the time.

We always say to our tutees: 'We don't mind if you don't work hard during your pre-reg year and don't pass your exam; we've done our pre-reg year, we've done our registration exam.' We think that whoever is looking after you in your rotations will have a similar view. It is not their responsibility to make sure that you learn from what you do. It's YOURS!

Until now you have probably only ever hung around with people whom you liked – it makes sense NOT to be with people whom you don't like. But, in a work environment, you may not have the opportunity to avoid people whom you do not like. It is hard, but you need to learn the art of working with people with whom you do not get on. So just bear in mind that you may not like everybody with whom you work, and they may not necessarily like you either, but in a workplace there are jobs to be done and that is the most important thing.

You will be working in many different teams during your pre-reg training year, so you need to develop some team-working skills. At first, it is likely that you will be treated as the most junior member of staff – as you probably know the least! As the training year progresses, your role will constantly change so that, by the end of the year, your role in the pharmacy team is significantly different to that at the start of the year. You will make that transition from student to professional, from trainee to pharmacist.

Bear in mind that it is not just pharmacists who work in a pharmacy or in a hospital. Try not to have any preconceived ideas as to what role befits different people – you will be surprised! And you will find that you are managed by technicians and assistants on a daily basis.

WHAT IS CLINICAL PHARMACY AND WHERE DOES IT HAPPEN?

One final point about 'clinical pharmacy': spending time on wards does not necessarily guarantee that you are doing 'clinical pharmacy'. What is this 'clinical pharmacy' and what does it mean to be a clinical pharmacist? We believe that ALL pharmacy is clinical pharmacy, whether you are on the wards or working in distribution, or anywhere else. Clinical pharmacy happens in a person's head – it is the thought behind what you are doing. This means that every pharmacist is a clinical pharmacist, whatever sector he or she is working in, and whatever setting he or she is practising in. Make sure that, wherever you are and whatever you are doing, you are training yourself to be a 'clinical pharmacist'.

'In my first rotation, the staff expected a lot from me right from the very beginning. Maybe staff should have lower expectations if pre-regs are going there for first rotation and the first week should be orientation, and there should be no unsupervised working in the first part of the rotation.'

'There were uncertain expectations in my first rotation. The first week I was shown things, and then in the second week I was doing everything which was actually a very steep learning curve!'

'My first rotation was on the surgical wards. It was a brilliant rotation; I really enjoyed it. I went in thinking that it was going to be crap – they only know how to cut things out, but they don't know about medicines, so I felt like I made quite a lot of input, which was good.'

TOP TIPS

- Being thrown in at the deep end can be an opportunity to show what you can do
- You are paid a decent salary; make sure that you earn it
- The pre-reg year is part of your professional training
- Think about what you consider as a professional and where you are now
- Manage your expectations in terms of what you want and what your employer can provide

---

REFERENCE

Stern DT. *Measuring Medical Professionalism.* Oxford: Oxford University Press, 2006.

Induction: getting to know your workplace and your team

2

Before you are due to start, make sure that you know some essential things, such as where you should be and when. In some hospitals all new starters are required to attend some kind of trust corporate induction, which can last for days. This trust induction may be held somewhere different to where you actually work, so please make sure that you turn up at the right place.

Make sure that you sort out anything that needs sorting before you start – for instance, you may need to bring with you important documentation such as degree certificates, passports or birth certificates. These can be hidden in all sorts of places and may need to be found in a box in a loft or somewhere similar! Or, if you cannot find them, you need to have looked in plenty of time so, if it can't be found, you have enough time to order a new one. If you need accommodation obviously you need to make sure that this is sorted out before you get there, otherwise you will have an incredibly stressful first few days. The most important of these is probably your proof of identity, and your bank and national insurance details, because without them there is little chance that you will get paid your first salary on time! When you turn up for the start of your placement, you will be required to fill out lots of paperwork, so make sure that you have the relevant documents with you. The human resources department need to process your documents, which is likely to be time-consuming and boring. It is necessary to ensure that you get the right contract of employment and to make sure that you get paid correctly.

It is useful to turn up with three vital pieces of equipment: a diary, a notebook and a pen that works. You will probably be told a great many things, most of which you will instantly forget! So be prepared to put appointments in your diary and write important things in your notebook. This means that you appear to be organised (even if you're are not naturally so).

On day 1, you will obviously be very nervous. You will be introduced to an entirely new workplace and to people with whom you will be working. The first day will be a whirlwind of a tour, most of which you will forget.

You will be working in an unfamiliar environment, carrying out tasks that you don't quite know how to do. This is all to be expected, so don't feel too downhearted. You may have some expectations of what you will be doing, and those expectations will probably turn out not to be true.

'Am feeling out of my comfort zone at the moment. . . . Not fully settled in. I feel weak. . . . I want to get the most out of this year.'

'The first month is hard. London is big. Not even time enough to settle in. My advice may be to move in the week before. I'm only just getting used to things. I find it hard to balance work, studying and life!'

'It takes 3 weeks to settle in – before you can move on. It is hard to be in an unknown environment. It makes me realise how little I know. I feel lucky that I have got friends here in London already.'

At this point in time, it is useful to get to know your fellow pre-regs and the people with whom you will be working. Surprisingly, this initial period may be one of the only times in your pre-reg training that you get to interact with your fellow pre-regs as a group, irrespective of whether there are only a few of you, or a whole gang. Once you start your rotations, you will be either working closely with one or two other pre-regs in each rotation, or by yourself. If you build up a good relationship with the other pre-regs right from the start, when you are split up into your different rotations you will know each other well enough to be able to ask each other for help and support.

'The first week was really good. It gave the pre-regs the opportunity to spend time with each other, which helps now. Would have taken a long time to get to know each other one by one. We help each other more now because we know each other. It was a very useful week – we may not have learnt much but we needed to set out standards of behaviour, etc.'

'I think I'm doing ok. It's been an emotional week. In general, I'm settling in well. We went out on Friday night, went out and got on really well, felt really happy. Most of us have bonded really well.'

Your pre-reg tutor is a very important person to you. He or she is the person who ultimately makes the decision – after discussion with you of course – as to whether or not to sign on the dotted line to say that you are competent and that you can be entered for the RPSGB registration examination at the end of your pre-reg training time. This means that it is vital for you to establish a good relationship with your tutor. Be careful not to get on his or her wrong side, otherwise you may find it difficult both to discuss any problems with the tutor and to get performance standards signed off. You do not want to be in a position towards the end of the year where you are having difficult discussions on whether you are competent, especially with someone with whom you have not got on very well.

You need to find out how your tutor works so that you can present yourself to him or her in the best possible light. Not all tutors are friendly and approachable; your tutor may be scary and unapproachable. You need to find this, and other things, out as soon as possible so that, when the time comes for formal progress reviews, you know how best to approach your tutor.

If your tutor is approachable, friendly and relaxed, hopefully this allows you to be the same. It is hoped that a friendly tutor is someone whom you can get to know well and with whom you can work well. But be careful; although you may find that you spend social time with your tutor, the tutor–tutee relationship is always an unequal relationship, and friendships cannot be fostered until your training year is over because your tutor has to maintain distance and be objective, as well as having the right to discipline you. We have always told our tutees that during their pre-reg year we are friendly with them, and may go out drinking and for meals with them, but that we cannot really be friends with them until they are qualified pharmacists.

If your tutor is unapproachable and unfriendly, you may have a bit of a battle on your hands. You, at first, need to establish what type of relationship you want to have with your tutor. Unfortunately you still have to work with him or her, and it is a good lesson to learn that not all the people with whom you work will like you, and vice versa. If you cannot get support from your tutor, you may have to find support from other sources such as fellow pre-regs or other pharmacists in your workplace to whom you can talk freely. The regional pharmacy teams and the pre-reg team at the RPSGB are useful, neutral and independent people with whom to talk if you have no one else.

It is definitely worth making an effort to get to know your tutor as early as possible. Find out what he or she requires from you in terms of evidence. Make an effort to provide enough evidence to demonstrate all your performance standards throughout your training period. Give your tutor every reason to sign you off. Also, bear in mind that your tutor is the person looking after you academically, and may not be your line manager. This means that you may need to report to different people for different things, which can become confusing.

'We now don't see our tutors in an ivory tower; now we can speak to tutors like normal. Induction gave us time so that we can see tutors are human beings.'

'We also got to know the tutors well during induction – they became more approachable and therefore more helpful.'

The other important person in your year is your pre-registration manager; this person may double up as a pre-reg tutor or be someone senior such as the chief pharmacist, but not a pre-reg tutor. The pre-reg manager is someone who is ultimately accountable to the RPSGB for the quality of the pre-reg training in that organisation.

In most hospitals, your first introduction to your workplace is through an induction period during which you are shown many different areas and meet many new people. In some places your induction is very short but in others (especially if they are a large pharmacy department) it may last for weeks. Don't expect to be doing much in your induction; the point is that you are being shown things and so you do not encounter very many opportunities where you can demonstrate anything competently!

The point of the induction is to familiarise you with your workplace and your work colleagues and, if you are one of many pre-regs, with your fellow pre-regs. Although it may not seem like you are doing very much in your induction, your managers are thinking about ensuring that you settle in and that the pre-regs can work together as a team. The more settled you feel, the easier you will find the year. You will have plenty of time in your rotations to demonstrate your competence, so enjoy the induction; it may be the only time during the year when you can be relatively relaxed!

'I knew that I wouldn't fully understand what pharmacists do still. It was a big reminder of how much I still need to learn. After the first teaching session, I went away with palpitations because I didn't know anything. It hit home that I needed to start to work.'

'I really liked the induction. It was a very good introduction to all the different areas. The first week was excellent. I was very nervous, being in a big hospital. It was a good transition between uni and work. I was ready to start work after induction.'

'I liked the induction – it meant that when I started my first rotation I was settled and calmer. It was a good opportunity for the whole team to bond, to get to know each other and understand each other. I had a problem with the initial week with getting frustrated; I was ready to go and do things, so I had to slow down.'

Before you even start to think about all the things that you need to achieve during your pre-reg training, you first need to get to know your workplace. Needless to say, it is very useful to become familiar with the layout of the hospital. Hospitals vary immensely in size, and in the ease with which you find your way around. Generally, the older the hospital, the more difficult it is to find your way around, and you may find yourself on a half-hour detour as you suddenly find yourself somewhere you've never been before. In your first few weeks, it is definitely worth familiarising yourself with your surroundings during a break or a lunchtime – if not for yourself, then for the patients who will be asking you, as an official-looking member of staff, for directions. Find out some important things, such as where to eat and drink, and alternative entrances and exits to the pharmacy department and the hospital.

'For the first week we met everybody, and that was really nice. We played games to get to know each other. This was really good because everyone was really scared. Too scared before this to do anything productive or learn anything new – the icebreakers made it easier.

'The clinical induction was useful to refresh my memory, to familiarise myself with the drug charts. I didn't take any drug histories. I have not taken a drug history as yet. It was more of a refresher of being on ward, learning what the standards are here. In the dispensary induction, it was useful to see where stuff was. We got to know where the basics were. This prepared me for my dispensary rotation. MI induction was good. It was useful to see the resources and to learn how other people did things and answer questions. Some activities seemed ridiculous at first, but it does come up. It was a good chance to get to know everyone. We were forced to get on with people that we did not know, to get to know each other better.'

Please bear in mind that you will be working in a pharmacy department and there are security issues with this. Although it may not be obvious to you, the pharmacy department is a highly sought-after destination for people who may want to get into the department and remove items. This means that, as an employee, you have a duty to uphold the security of the department, which means wearing and displaying your own ID badge at all times (which you should have received when you first start) and reporting your lost ID badge if it is ever lost or stolen. In addition, whenever you enter or leave the department, be careful for whom you are holding the door open – if you do not know who the person is you need to challenge him or her. If an unknown person gains entry to the pharmacy department there are implications in terms of the safety and security of the staff and the products held securely inside the department.

Get to know the people with whom you are to work. It is likely that you will be introduced to a vast number of new faces at the start, and you will probably forget many. Try to be as friendly and open as possible and not too overwhelmed. You will meet a whole range of pharmacy and non-pharmacy staff in those initial days. Other than fellow pre-regs, your closest colleagues will be newly qualified pharmacists. You are probably in awe of these newly qualified pharmacists, but remember that, a year ago, they were where you are now, and they have been qualified as pharmacists only for a few weeks at the most. They look like they know what they are doing, but believe us when we say that they are as scared as you are – probably more so. There will also be a whole raft of other people with whom you are to work. Try not to have any preconceived ideas about what pharmacists, technicians and assistants do, because you will probably be proved wrong.

Another thing to think about is the fact that you are not the only 'student' group in the hospital requiring training. You are fighting for training with other student groups such as pre-registration trainee pharmacy technicians (student technicians) and rotational staff rotating through the area that you are in. Remember that the onus is on you to direct your training and to make the most of your training experiences, so you may need to be assertive at times because pre-reg training is not uppermost in most people's minds. Those of you who have had some work experience in hospital pharmacies may have experienced this already.

Try to join in with any social activities that are planned, however daunting this may be to a new starter like yourself! You will generally find that it is easier to work with people if you have socialised with them on some level outside work, although bear in mind that, if you do socialise with work mates, you should avoid doing anything too embarrassing because you have to face everyone at work the next day and may have given a bad first impression of yourself!

When you start your training, you are provided with RPSGB pre-registration training folders. Do yourself a favour and read through them! These folders contain almost everything that there is to know about the year and have some useful activities for you to do as you go through the year. They contain official paperwork, such as the learning contract and the progress reviews, as well as the pre-registration training byelaws; for those of you who like to test yourselves they also have a sample registration exam paper. The earlier that you get to grips with what is required, the earlier you can start to demonstrate to your tutor that you are competent.

Please be aware that much c towards single community pharma thought many of the preparatory e instance, you probably do not need you need to do to show compete because it is likely that, in a hospi different sections of pharmacy ea performance standards while perfc tion, your tutor should make it clea pay particular attention.

Every hospital trust is part of required to attend regional study d have some study days away from complement your work-based trainii out throughout the pre-registration t specific programme. Please note that in which the study days happen may undertake your rotations, but pay cl learning in the regional study days s

Use the regional study days to other hospitals, and to meet up with are good for networking and compa with what others are doing in other h find that your experience in your ho other pre-regs in other hospital sites some comfort in the fact that you are difficulties wherever you are doing y

---

TOP TIPS

- Make a good first impression
- Expect a lot of paperwork, ru period
- Make an effort to get to kno makes your life easier
- Meet with your tutor and dor

Please be aware that much of the information in the folder is geared towards single community pharmacist pre-reg tutors. Your tutor will have thought many of the preparatory exercises through before you get there. For instance, you probably do not need to think too much about what activities you need to do to show competency in certain performance standards, because it is likely that, in a hospital environment, your rotations through different sections of pharmacy easily allow you to demonstrate different performance standards while performing particular duties. During induction, your tutor should make it clear to what parts of the folder you should pay particular attention.

Every hospital trust is part of a pre-registration region and you will be required to attend regional study days. These are an opportunity for you to have some study days away from your workplace on subject areas that complement your work-based training. These study days are generally spread out throughout the pre-registration training year and every region has its own specific programme. Please note that, as the programme is regional, the order in which the study days happen may not coincide with the order in which you undertake your rotations, but pay close attention, because sooner or later the learning in the regional study days should become useful to you.

Use the regional study days to make friends with other pre-regs from other hospitals, and to meet up with your university friends. These study days are good for networking and comparing and contrasting what you are doing with what others are doing in other hospitals. This may give you a voice if you find that your experience in your hospital does not compare well with what other pre-regs in other hospital sites are doing. On the flipside, you may take some comfort in the fact that you are all in the same boat and have the same difficulties wherever you are doing your training.

TOP TIPS

- Make a good first impression by being prepared
- Expect a lot of paperwork, rules and regulations in your induction period
- Make an effort to get to know your team and your workplace; it makes your life easier
- Meet with your tutor and don't be scared!

The pre-reg team – team dynamics

3

YOU, THE PRE-REGS AND THE WORKING TEAM

You will generally be with more than one pre-reg in your training programme because it is very rare for hospitals to offer pre-reg places for one person only. You may be in a team of just 2 pre-regs or you may have up to 15 others in your team in a larger hospital; generally teaching hospitals tend to take more pre-regs. Even if you are in a small team, you will be working as part of a larger team in the rotation or area in which you are working, so it is important that you understand how group, or team, dynamics can have an influence on you or how you may be influencing the dynamics, even inadvertently.

It is very important that you get to know the other members of your team because you will be spending the year together and may well be leaning on each other in times of difficulty. You may never have worked closely with others during your university days where there is often competition among students, and the type of work and experiences that you may be sharing during pre-reg are probably things that you have never experienced before. In rotations, you will be working with the same people for a number of weeks.

Before you get to know your team, and two people are still a team, it is important that you get to know yourself first because, if there are any problems during the year, they may well be problems relating to you. You need to identify how well you work in a team, what really makes you enjoy the team working aspect and what you really hate when working as part of a team. You may well have said that you enjoy team working in your application form for pre-reg, and said the same during your interview, but the question is: Did you really mean it? A lot of people think that the 'best' role within a team is to be the leader, but this is not always the case and there can be too many leaders in any one team, resulting in conflicts and disagreements.

Some people are natural team players and others are not, however much they pretend that they are. It is important that you identify this for yourself because there is no doubt that, if you are not that good in a team, you will be found out over the course of the year when the pressure is on. You may want to ask yourself the following questions:

- What do I really like when I am part of a team?
- What role do I prefer in a team?
- How do I feel when someone else has taken up the role that I usually have?
- Do I need to compete to regain my role or am I content to let someone else have the same role as me?
- What do I dislike about being in a team?
- How much individual freedom can I have to do my own thing?

Although these questions are not exhaustive, and certainly not questions that you necessarily need to share with anyone else, they are worth asking.

There may be occasions over the course of the year when you find yourself becoming distant from the team and wanting your own freedom to do your own thing without always having to join the group and be a part of it. Some of you may not be able to relate to this but others will. It can be difficult to exclude yourself when you have generally been an active part of the group. In any team, there is a commitment to work together at the start of the year or rotation and, as time progresses, you may find that you need your own direction. This is more likely to happen if you are in a smaller team because you may be the exact opposite to the rest of the team. An example is when the team go out socialising; you may not want to go with them because they go out drinking and drinking is not your thing. How are you going to exclude yourself from this without damaging any relationship that you have built with your team? It may be that you do not care much about these relationships because you are in it only for yourself, and you have no interest in maintaining friendships after the pre-reg year. This is perfectly OK but be prepared for the team to move on to other things without you if you are in a minority. This is much less of a problem in a larger team because you are more likely to find others to whom you can relate; larger hospitals have more pharmacy staff, so you will generally find someone you like, even if they are not a pre-reg.

In a smaller hospital you may find that you prefer the company of other hospital staff or people with whom you are living if you are away from the family home. If you live with your parents, you always have your family and own circle of friends as well as mates from uni.

WHAT MAKES A TEAM?

There is a plethora of literature about teams and what makes a good team in management books; we do not deal with this here because it is outside of the scope of this book. We have intentionally avoided trying to identify a list of qualities that make a good team because of the ready availability in existing literature.

It is important at this stage to identify the difference between a group and a team. A group is a collection of individuals who are gathered together and associate themselves with each other – this is what a pre-reg group will be like at the start of the year. A group in itself does not necessarily constitute a team. Teams normally have members with complementary skills, generating synergy through a coordinated effort; this allows each member to maximise his or her strengths and minimise his or her weaknesses. A team is a group of people with a common purpose.

From our point of view, as pre-reg tutors and managers, a good pre-reg team is a bonus because there could be a better collective group effort. If pre-regs do not form a team this does not affect how we do our jobs and support pre-regs; we continue to support pre-regs individually regardless, but this may be more difficult.

An analogy that we often use is trying to relate the pre-reg team to a sports team such as football and netball. Using the football analogy, a good team is one in which the team members have different sets of skill which they combine to maximise the team effort. You do not find more than one goalkeeper in a football team (assuming no substitutes of course!). Problems may occur if there are more than two strikers on the team and they do not complement each other; in these instances conflict may arise when they both want the limelight and are not prepared to put in the effort required when working in a team, such as defending and chasing back.

The same can be said about the team in netball which has only seven players on each team. The ball cannot be passed from the goal defence to the goal shooter unless it has passed through at least one team member. As netball rules do not permit players to take more than one step in possession of the ball, the only way to move the ball towards the goal is to throw the ball to a team mate. The ball cannot be held by a player for more than 3 seconds at any time, which ensures that everyone on the team is regularly involved in play. If one player does not play her part in the team the whole team will be unsuccessful because the ball will not get from one end of the court to the other.

Although the sporting analogy will not suit all of you, when it comes to trying to describe the advantages of a good team many will relate to this straight away.

In larger pre-reg teams the team members all have slightly different qualities; in those teams that work well, pre-regs have maximised the benefit of working in the team by identifying each other's strengths and weaknesses. An example is where those of you who are good at calculations may be called upon to help the weaker ones to do calculations, and in return you may benefit from sharing their knowledge and experience. There is a similar situation in rotational teams but it may take longer to establish the roles of the individual players and your own role within that team. You don't want to be the one who is always offside or always dropping the ball at important moments!

While considering what makes a good team, it is equally important to think about either what makes a bad team or how a good team becomes a bad one. A bad team is one in which the members break into smaller groups; this often happens in teams with more than five or six members, and the two or more groups completely divorce themselves from each other. Each small group has its own identity and direction and they often socialise together both in and out of work. There are occasions when the smaller groups are so dissimilar that conflict can develop. This is seen particularly when the pre-reg year becomes stressful, such as around recruitment time and in the build-up to the registration exam. A good team can easily break down into smaller groups and, although this is normal, the team should still be able to function as a whole when there is a common goal.

We sometimes see individuals excluded from the main team, for whatever reason, and they have to 'go it alone' during the year. For some of you this may be OK but for others this can be distressing and add to the stress already there, particularly during group activities.

Another way to look at the team is to think of the members differently:

- Players: make it (make things happen); these are the people who embrace the workload and are actively involved in what is going on. They will often make sacrifices in their own work for the benefit of the team. These are obviously the best types of people to work with and it would be good if you were an active player in any team in which you work.
- Spectators: hope it and want it (don't like change and can be cynical); these are the people who like to sit on the outside; they work hard and have opinions on what is going on, but don't like to get involved too much. They are happy just doing the work required of them and then going home.

• Corpses: no idea, don't care (have always done it like this); these people may not care so much about the workplace and have no idea what is happening in the department or the profession in terms of developments. They are just there to do their jobs. They will be the ones who do not read the *Pharmaceutical Journal* or keep themselves up to date, and you may feel somewhat demoralised working alongside them. Trust us; these people do exist!

• Terrorists: stop it (tend to respond to people who are always negative and challenging); these people are generally resistant to change and have always done things a certain way. They won't take kindly to your well-intentioned suggestions of changing anything. They usually work behind the scenes and are very negative; they may 'use' you in their game to prevent something from happening and it is worth watching out for anything out of the ordinary with which you find yourself getting involved. Remember that in any department there are always politics of some sort going on.

GROUP DYNAMICS AND THE PRE-REG YEAR

There are many theories relating to group dynamics in the management literature but one theory that sits comfortably in the pre-reg year relates to the stages of group formation and how groups go through the same stages.

Bruce Tuckman (1965) proposed a model, known as Tuckman's stages, for a group. Tuckman's model states that the ideal group decision-making process should occur in five stages and this is how groups, e.g. a pre-reg group, may function:

• Forming
• Storming
• Norming
• Performing
• Mourning.

It should be noted that this model refers to the overall pattern of the group, although individuals within a group work in different ways and may not go through the stages at the same rate as the whole group. If distrust persists, a group may never even get to the norming stage, remaining stuck in perpetual conflict in the storming stage. Although the explanations below refer mainly to a large pre-reg team, they are equally applicable to working teams in rotations, e.g. the dispensary, although the stages of group formation may progress quicker or get stuck at a particular stage because rotations are generally only for a few weeks.

Forming

This is the first stage of any group formation. At the start of the pre-reg year, during induction, you will all be trying to get to know each other and get along with each other. Some hospitals have an induction period for you to get to know each other better, as well as for getting used to the new working environment. This stage is sometimes known as the 'honeymoon phase' in which everyone is just trying to get along, with any differences in personalities being swept under the carpet. Everyone is nice and polite with each other, even if the behaviour and opinions of others differ significantly. The group is starting to form and, as time progresses, you will start to identify the characteristics of the other pre-regs. Sometimes this stage is quite quick and, by the end of the induction period, if you have one, the gloves are off and there is some movement and jostling among group members as you all try to find people with whom you will get along and share interests.

This can be a tricky stage for the pre-reg group because you may have other pre-regs in your group who were your friends at university or went to the same university as you. You may find yourself going towards such pre-regs because this is the only common ground that you have; you may not have spoken to the others while at university because you had different circles of friends. On the other hand, you may be the only one from your university and find it rather difficult to break into a group who all know each other from previously.

The other difficulty is that you may not be a very confident person and need some time to get to know people; you may not feel comfortable approaching people whom you do not know. Hopefully others in the group will make this easier for you by trying to get to know you, so that you do not need to make the first move. This stage can be similar to starting a new school, college or university, when you had to get to know your classmates; the only difference is that now you will be together in a work environment for a year.

'We have had a good chance to get to know everyone. At first, we were all split into two groups, but this broke down at end of induction, which may not have happened if induction had not happened. We were forced to get on with people that we may not know, to get to know each other better.'

'I don't think that I have socially fitted in well because I am never here. There are a lot of people with personalities, and I'm not really getting involved in that.'

'Everyone is so different.'

Storming

The next stage can be either problematic for the group or fairly straightforward; this depends on your relationships with the rest of the pre-regs. Some of you may find that this stage has gone quickly and smoothly because relationships have been established and everyone is happy with them. Others may find that this is the most difficult stage but did not want to speak up and say something for the sake of the group. This could happen because you are a quiet person and as a result the others have labelled you in a particular way and not involved you, so you end up with a certain role in the group. This stage could be difficult if you were used to being one of the leaders and the centre of attention at 'home' or university, when now you are faced with a situation where you have to compete with other pre-regs whom you do not know. This may take the form of disagreements over a range of things, from how to undertake a particular task at work to where to go out with the pre-reg group.

The honeymoon phase is well and truly over and the true personalities are beginning to come through as people seek to establish themselves. Sometimes this can bring out the worst in you and, on occasions, you may not even be aware of this yourself. All pretence of being polite to each other has been dropped and tempers can often flare up. A particular difficulty can be where the pre-reg group is imbalanced in terms of males and females, with more females in the group. This is generally the balance in hospital pharmacy where women outnumber men.

You may feel that you are being victimised and perhaps even bullied by other members of the group, and have to go along with decisions being made by the majority. You have to decide whether you can be flexible and join them – if you can't beat them, join them – or whether you are happy doing your own thing. In our experience, there have been occasions when two pre-regs who were previously friends from the same university had a complete breakdown of their relationship, with the result that they could not be in the same room together let alone undertake group tasks. This can sometimes cause the group to fracture and become two distinct, mutually exclusive groups. Other examples are where an individual has arrived in a group that was already formed, e.g. for sandwich course placements, which has disrupted the group with the result that new groups formed. We discuss the experiences of sandwich course placements elsewhere in the book.

During this stage the group starts to establish roles: there are some leaders, some followers and some general group members, and a team starts to form. Referring to the team, some prefer to take up the striker, or goal shooter, role whereas others prefer to act for the defence, leaving the general team players as the midfield. As the group identifies individuals' strengths and weaknesses a team purpose starts to develop. On occasions a hierarchy may develop in which certain people are looked up to within the team, playing the role of team captain, but generally a team of 'equals' means that there is flexibility for the range of tasks and situations encountered during the pre-reg year.

Norming

This stage follows the storming stage and is where the team starts to get used to each other and members are happy to disclose their strengths and weaknesses for the benefit of the team. The team are getting used to each other's company and there is no pressure from the other pre-regs to always be a part of the team. There is more honesty and openness and, if you do not want to get involved in a particular activity, this is accepted by the others. This stage is quite nice because things have moved on from the conflict stage; if two people do not get on with each other, this is recognised, sometimes implicitly, and the two keep away from each other or are polite towards each other without being the best of friends. This is important in any size of pre-reg group because, if there are only two of you, you will either just do your own thing or work together; in larger groups, smaller subgroups begin to develop but the group as a whole still functions as a team.

'I think I'm ok. It's getting better. The first few weeks I felt like I was different, thinking wise and character wise. I am a bit more used to the dynamic now and feel more comfortable. We are now doing so much social activities, which I find surprising. It is good when we are in a big group and all go for lunch.'

Performing

This is the best stage of any group or team and is where you all work well together with a common purpose and dedication. All know their roles and are comfortable with them, and work is shared among the team, with everyone helping each other out. Although we all hope that this stage is prolonged over the year, in actual fact the group can go backwards and forwards from this stage as the pre-reg year progresses and brings different challenges. Towards the end of the year, when preparation for the registration exam is at its height, if the team is at the performance stage then everyone is helping each other out with revision and help, support and guidance.

This stage can be encountered earlier on in the year when, in larger groups, a group task is given to you and you have to work together to achieve this. An example of this is if you have been allocated the task to arrange a departmental party, such as the Christmas party, which is traditional in some hospitals. The group then becomes a team and you work together to make sure that the party is a success; this can occur even if the group is going through the storming or norming stages.

> 'I think that I fit in. I realise that I am starting to withdraw into myself. I like to be by myself. This must be a symptom of being an only child. I enjoy the dynamics of the team. Initially everybody thought we had to be best friends but now we've realised that's not possible. I'm having fun – and I've learnt times to be quiet in a group situation. Everything's going well.'
>
> 'There are a few of us from the same uni, but we were not all close when we were there. I would like to think that I fit in with everybody but there is one person that I just don't get on with as much. But working with them will be fine.'

Mourning

Although it is obvious that this stage occurs at the end of the lifecycle of a group, there are other times in the year when this can also occur. The turn of the calendar year is when the recruitment for pharmacist positions usually occurs and it is sometimes at this stage that the team re-forms and goes through the stages again.

You may find that you are competing with your peers for the same jobs in your hospital, which may cause some friction and conflict because this may be the first time that you are in direct competition with each other. This can be considered as the storming stage revisited and the group quickly goes through the other stages to the mourning stage once the winners and losers have been identified. Sometimes the pre-reg team can break down into those who have got the jobs that they wanted and those who still have to be successful in the jobs that they want. If you are one of the lucky ones who have got the job of your choice, you can sometimes find it difficult to stay within the team as it was before because you may feel guilty about being successful at the expense of your peers, some of whom you may think were better candidates than you. Alternatively, you may feel the opposite and start to move away from the team and look towards the people with whom you may be working once you have qualified. This may well alienate you from the rest of the pre-reg team. It will mark the end of the pre-reg team and be a watershed moment; it is interesting to see how you all react and behave towards each other during the time of recruitment.

The other time that this stage is encountered is at the end of the training year, when you get your registration exam results. Most pre-reg years finish very soon after the exam results; some years finish on the day of the results, so that you have very little time to absorb the enormity of passing the exam and then saying goodbye to the pre-reg team. There will be some sort of gathering when you may all be together at the end of the year, although this does not always happen; in some instances you may take the day off from work to get your results and never see each other in the pre-reg team ever again; although disappointing, this does happen.

You will all say that you will keep in touch with each other and with your tutors, but in reality it is very unlikely that you will stay in touch unless you have made real friendships during the year. In our experience, few pre-regs actually stay in touch with each other, or their tutors, after the pre-reg year; they move on to the next stages in their careers. Even if they see each other after the pre-reg year, it is never the same as it was during the year.

'We generally get on quite well. Generally everyone is really nice but there is a lot of pre-reg politics. There is someone that I don't really talk to. I try to avoid conflict and I can't put a finger on what the problem is.'

'I think I have settled in well. In terms of the pre-reg team, I felt a bit scared when I thought that everybody wanted to be friends. Then we split off into our own rotations – for me it's worked out fine. There have been some issues – of which I don't want to get involved, I'm just going to ignore it. I am slightly worried about some of the other pre-regs' relationships.'

'It's been a bit difficult since some of us have got jobs here and some have not. It makes it hard for you to get along. I thought that we were very close friends but it has made me realise that we have only known each other for a few months and that that is not long enough for us to be real friends if something like this is causing a problem.'

TOP TIPS

- There is no 'I' in team
- Establish your place in the team and be flexible
- Identify your strengths and weaknesses in the team
- Be honest to your team
- Try to find out more about the members of your team in terms of their team roles

---

REFERENCE

Tuckman B. Developmental sequence in small groups. *Psychological Bulletin* 1965; 63: 384–99.

Your tutor: developing that special relationship

4

GETTING TO KNOW YOUR TUTOR

The first time that you find out who your tutor is going to be is when you send in your RPSGB notification form to the hospital for the tutor and manager to complete, before it goes back to the RPSGB with your cheque for payment for the pre-reg year. At this point this is just a name on the form; you probably don't know who this person actually is.

At this stage it is well worth your effort to find out who your tutor is going to be in terms of his or her role within the pharmacy department at the hospital. You may even want to contact him or her beforehand to touch base and find out more. A word of caution, however; your tutor may turn out to be the chief pharmacist who is probably a very busy person. In some hospitals the role of the pre-reg tutor is taken very seriously and there are dedicated education and training pharmacists who undertake these roles; in other hospitals, while still being taken seriously, the pre-reg tutor is a pharmacist whose main role is in another area in the pharmacy and the role of the tutor is tagged onto their main role. There are advantages and disadvantages with each and, to be honest, it does not really matter because what you make of the year is up to you and your tutor is there to guide and support you.

Some hospitals try to have one tutor for each individual pre-reg so there can be quite a few pre-reg tutors at the hospital, depending on the size of the hospital, although they are generally overseen and supported by a pharmacist who has overall responsibility for pre-reg training; this is usually the pre-reg manager. Most pre-reg tutors, but by no means all, are quite senior pharmacists although it must be said that not all like, or are any good at, being tutors, and they have these responsibilities placed upon them by their seniors. These pharmacists may have little knowledge, or experience, of what the pre-reg programme involves and how to support you throughout the year. If you are unlucky enough to be one of the ones to have such a tutor, it is very important that you try to manage your own training year as much as you can. You must also make sure that you are completely familiar with the requirements of the training programme, so it is definitely worth reading through any documentation sent to you by the RPSGB.

Although most of you will know nothing about your tutors until you arrive, it may be worth asking your pharmacy friends or colleagues if you have heard anything about your new tutor. Pharmacy can be a very small world and you may be surprised when someone knows someone who knows of your tutor. Any information can be useful, particularly if you have colleagues who have completed, or are undertaking, their pre-reg year at the hospital to which you are going.

When you arrive at the hospital, you will no doubt meet your tutor at some point during the induction. It is important to make a good impression on the tutor as early as possible. For some of you, you may find that you do not actually meet your tutor until a few weeks into the year because they are on holiday or have other commitments. Remember that the pre-reg year starts in July or August, which is the time of summer holidays so most pharmacy departments are short staffed and very busy. You should meet somebody who is going to look after you and cover for your tutor, although this is unfortunately not always the case.

If your induction goes to plan, you meet the people who will be managing your pre-reg year and find out what the year will involve in terms of your rotations and on which hospital sites you will be working. You meet your pre-reg manager and, hopefully, your pre-reg tutor. This may be a bit scary at first, particularly if your tutor is the chief pharmacist of a very large hospital but you don't need to be scared because they are all human! It may be the case that your tutor is senior and many staff in the department either do not like, or are apprehensive of, him or her. This may be because your tutor is a senior manager and has to make decisions that are not popular. Remember that the face that the tutor shows to you may be very different from what he or she shows to the rest of the department – he or she is probably a nice person underneath the persona.

It is important to realise that your tutor is there to support you throughout the year and assess you against performance standards, but not do any of the work for you. Tutors do not have time to do this, and it is your pre-reg year after all. Some of you may expect them to be the fount of all knowledge and to be able to answer all your questions; you may therefore be disappointed to find that most tutors generally answer your questions with more questions although they may provide you with some direction as to where to find the answers. This could well be frustrating for some of you who expect answers to your questions; your tutors are not university lecturers. You may also find it frustrating when your tutor presents you with an ambiguous problem and asks you to find an answer or make a decision; you then find that there is more than one correct answer and that, although your answer is correct according to the literature or the books, it is not what your tutor would do. You should be able to discuss this with your tutor to see why he or she makes a particular decision.

You need to be aware of your own deadlines and when your rotations occur, and also what deadlines are set by the RPSGB for any formal documentation. You need to inform your tutor of these deadlines, if they are not already aware of them, so that you can work towards them. Some experienced tutors will guide you on this but do not expect guidance from all tutors.

MANAGING THE BOSS

We would recommend that, in your early meetings with your tutor, you try to find out a bit more about him or her in terms of what he or she does in the department and how his or her diary works. The more senior your tutor, the busier the diary will invariably be. It is important to find out the tutor's interests, for example respiratory medicine or pharmacokinetics, and then make sure that you revise these areas because it is likely that you will be asked questions about these areas in your tutor meetings. If your tutor is one of the senior managers, it is worth finding out how he or she would like to support you and how often he or she normally sees pre-regs during the year. If your tutor prefers you to come to him or her we recommend that you try to set up meetings in advance, in particular around the time that you finish your rotations and certainly around the time of the formal progress reviews. Tutors with the busier diaries may prefer this because they are then committed to seeing you at an allocated time; be aware that often their diaries will change and they may need to move any meetings with you. You need to make sure that you are organised and make a note of any changes to meetings in your own diary. On occasions you may find that your meetings are moved to a different time of the day, a different day or a different site; all of these changes can get very confusing.

Once you have established how your tutor is going to support you and how often you will meet, it is important that you manage this effectively throughout the year. Remember that your tutor will probably be so busy that if you do not see him or her then he or she will not see you. In our experience, if pre-regs do not try to make appointments with their tutors, they can go weeks without seeing them. When you do finally see your tutor, he or she may not have enough time to go through your records of evidence, and then at progress review time he or she will not have seen enough evidence to sign you off. It is important for you to realise that, without enough evidence, your tutor will not sign you off and it will be you who suffers because the tutor has nothing to lose.

Many hospital pre-reg tutors will not work with you directly during the year; some may work with you in particular rotations, and they need you to provide them with evidence of what you have been doing during the rotation. Remember that it is unlikely that your tutor is an expert in all pharmacy practice areas and you may well be teaching him or her new things that you have learned during your rotations. Conversely, you need to be honest with your tutors in areas in which you have little experience or at which you are just not very good. Once you have identified your weaknesses, it makes it much easier for you to strengthen these areas during the year. It pays in the long term for you to be honest and identify the real problems that you may have. For example, you may just not be very good at seeing patients with terminal illness and this is something that you may not feel comfortable about disclosing to anyone else. Your tutor will either be able to help you by providing his or her own experiences or may direct you to someone who may be able to help you more than he or she can; only a bad tutor will leave you in the lurch and not do anything. You need to communicate clearly with your tutor and be clear about any problems that you may have. Don't beat about the bush. You need to learn from your own experiences in the work-place but it is worth learning from your tutor's experience as well.

In these instances it is important to provide your tutor with appropriate evidence of what you have been doing. Most hospitals prefer you to use records of evidence and some hospitals have devised their own paperwork for this. You need to remember to provide copies of prescriptions, drug charts or documents to go with the records of evidence, so that your tutor knows that what you have done is genuine; without this there is no guarantee that your evidence is not fabricated. Often tutors will check with others in the department to see if what you are writing is a true reflection of what you have been doing, and whether any patients about whom you are writing are not actually in the hospital. It is not unheard of for pre-regs to write records of evidence that are not true accounts of what actually happened, and they claim that they did things that they did not.

It would be worth checking with your tutor how he or she prefers you to supply your records of evidence. Some tutors prefer to have these a few days before you are due to meet so that they can go through them before the meeting; others prefer to have them during the tutor meetings and then go through them during the meetings. Unless you are meeting your tutor for different reasons there is little point in attending a tutor meeting with no records of evidence and nothing to discuss. It is not uncommon for pre-regs to appear at a tutor meeting with nothing to discuss – the only reason their presence being because this was in their diary; this is very frustrating for the tutor and is a wasted meeting, so try to ensure that you do not do this. It is far better to postpone and reschedule your meeting.

Experienced tutors will be familiar with the requirements of the pre-reg in terms of the performance standards and will guide you when claiming for these standards in your records; some hospitals have developed their own guides to the performance standards. Other, less experienced, tutors will be less familiar with the standards and it may be up to you to ensure that what you are claiming for is actually appropriate. There is a lot of guidance in the RPSGB portfolios as they are set up in a way that provides activities for you to complete in preparation for tutor meetings and formal progress reviews; completing these activities may be very useful.

This is what the whole pre-reg year is based on and you need to make every learning opportunity count for something. Your tutor can help you in identifying learning opportunities and also provide you with support by seeing if your rotations can be changed or made longer if this is an identified area of weakness for you.

WHAT CAN GO WRONG?

There are many things that can go wrong with your tutor; some of them may be of your making and others may be outside your control but frustrating nevertheless.

It is absolutely critical that you start your year on a positive note, with the expectation that the pre-reg year is your year and that you are responsible for making sure that you cover everything that you need to cover.

From our experience, some things that can go wrong with your tutor, apart from the lack of experience and interest, include the following:

- Tutor too busy, e.g. may work part time
- Tutor leaves and no one available to cover
- Tutor goes on long-term leave, e.g. maternity leave, and no one to cover
- Tutor works on a different hospital site to you and is difficult to get hold of
- Tutor is unfriendly and unsupportive
- Tutor has too high expectations of you
- Work is too busy and you are not allowed to leave your rotation to see your tutor.

Some of the problems that are your fault include:

- You are consistently late and unprepared for your meetings
- You do not write sufficient quality records of evidence
- You do not show any development over a period of time
- You do not learn from your experiences
- You do not have an insight into your own weaknesses
- You do not recognise your own limitations
- You do not respond well to criticism.

In our experience some or all of the above have happened and are sometimes difficult to manage. Many of these problems can be resolved by good communication with your tutors at the start of the year, but occasionally it is difficult to do this, especially if your tutor is a senior pharmacist. Our advice is that, if there are any problems with your tutor, take these up with your pre-reg manager who is ultimately accountable for pre-reg training in the hospital. You will find that the pre-reg manager will generally be interested to hear your views and may even be able to change your tutor midway through the year, if you both feel that the relationship is not working. If your pre-reg tutor is also the pre-reg manager, you may want to go to his or her manager, but take a look at yourself first in case any of the problems are of your own making and try to resolve these first.

If your tutor is your manager and also the chief pharmacist, you have a problem! In these cases, it is worth noting that help and support are available from outside the hospital. Every hospital will be part of a region and you will have regional study days, so you may want to discuss any issues with the regional team who are neutral to the hospital and will try to support you by listening to you and providing you with advice in a confidential manner. Other than that, the pre-reg team at the RPSGB are very experienced at handling pre-reg problems; although contacting the professional body can be daunting, it is still an option.

TOP TIPS

- Identify your tutor's job, roles and responsibilities
- Get to know your tutor and how he or she works
- Learn how to organise yourself and your tutor
- Never arrive at tutor meetings with nothing done or nothing to discuss
- Have opinions on your own progress and be honest

5

Making the transition from student to professional: how to get through the year

When you first arrive in your pre-reg placement, you are very much the student because, although some of you may have experienced pharmacy practice, you will not have done this from the viewpoint of a pharmacist. All that knowledge that you got from your university degree will need to be applied in practice and the pre-reg year is the time to do this.

What do we mean by a student? Well, for many pre-regs, just coming to work every day is something that they have never done before. We realise that many of you will have done some part-time work or even worked full time for a short time, but working, learning and being assessed all at the same time is not that easy. We have experienced a whole range of pre-regs from those who take to their training programme like a fish to water to those who struggle for some time to break out of that student mentality. Those pre-regs who struggle often do so because they expect their trainers and tutors to provide them with lots of direction, i.e. tell them what to do, and they tend to expect too much – in a sense they will always be in training rather than contributing to the service needs of the department. As we have said before, you are paid a decent salary to be a pre-reg so you need to give something back to the department. There will be times when you will be asked to do things that you consider to be boring or beneath your role as a pre-reg. Get over it! You are there to work first and foremost, and the training or experience comes from this. If you embrace these opportunities and use them to gain more experience, you will have a much better idea of what is involved. Some pre-regs think that they are only there to learn and develop in the things that they want to do, with no regard for what the service needs. In many hospitals, you may be pulled out of whichever rotation you are in and asked to come and help, for example, in the dispensary. If this is the case, take a look around and see why you have been asked to help; it will probably be because they are busy.

'At first, when I started, my most difficult experience was with patient contact. After watching other pre-regs talk to patients, there was no choice, so I just had to get on with it.'

'At the beginning the technicians and pharmacists expected a lot right from the beginning. Maybe staff should have lower expectations of pre-regs going there for their first rotation with no unsupervised working in first part of rotation.'

'I think there should be more support in the first rotation.'

'At the beginning, we were made to feel less than what we are – but thinking about it now, we are at the bottom.'

'My supervisor was not around at first, so I had to report to someone else. It was a bit difficult in this rotation. You had to stand back to let others get on with things – and you were trying to find things to do, and also not really reporting to anyone. I didn't know whom to ask, and I was trying to find things to do. I felt like a burden. It was difficult and I was getting in trouble by talking too much.'

Your progress in the training year can be like completing a jigsaw puzzle, except that you do not necessarily know what the final puzzle looks like. At the start of the year it is as if you have been given a box with puzzle pieces and told to go away and start putting the puzzle together. You do not know where to start!

As your training programme progresses you will find that you are progressing and seeing things in a different way. What you have learned at university is important but you start to realise that there is no textbook patient and what you have learned is not as black and white as you thought. Many pre-regs initially struggle with this; there is often more than one correct answer. An example to illustrate this is a patient who has co-morbidities such as heart failure, respiratory disease and renal failure. At university you may have learned abut these in separate modules and may know how to manage each of these conditions separately, whereas in the real world one patient can have all of these conditions with one possibly affecting the other. This is why it is important to bring all the knowledge together and think wider than the individual problems. Add to this the patient who does not believe in his or her medicines and does not adhere/comply, and the problem is wider than at first sight.

The first few months of the training programme can be very intense and it is not unusual to think that you did not learn anything useful at university; this of course is not the case because, otherwise, how did you get through?

You will often be very tired at the end of the working week because everyone is giving you extra tasks to do and you have to learn about such things as drugs and conditions about which you know nothing. Even if you are in a rotation that you do not like, you will find that there are things for you to learn. Pre-regs who have a student mentality may expect people to provide work and not think in terms of what extra contribution they could make. They sit there and expect someone to come and speak to them and tell them what to do next. Guess what, that is not going to happen in a busy working environment. The same pre-regs often complain to their tutors that they did not benefit from that particular rotation. This is not to say that there are no difficult rotations, just that you make what you want of your pre-reg time.

'I've changed since starting here – I feel like I've finally grown up. I've learnt a lot in certain ways, I've learnt a lot about work life. The biggest change has been that everything you learnt at uni is used but not in the way I thought it would be used. I do not know anything at work and I'm still asking silly questions and doing silly things. As a person, I need to improve by being a bit more open, to try to think where to look rather than ask questions all the time. To try to do things by myself.'

'I was thrown in at deep end. The first few days, I saw what my supervisor did to ease into things. Then I started to do drug histories myself. Then I progressed with problems and making recommendations to doctors. Towards the end of this first rotation, I could go up on my own and do drug histories and get information, and I was itching for more.'

'In terms of making decisions, I feel very protected. I'm not allowed to do anything without supervision. I'm from a community background where I had some autonomy so I am finding this supervision smothering already. At the moment, everything I have learnt is textbook knowledge and it is hard to apply everything in practice.'

By the middle of the pre-reg year, you will have started to work out your own way of completing the puzzle. Some pre-regs start at the middle and build up a picture, whereas others will find the pieces around the edges and start putting these together. In this way you start to identify the shape and dimensions of the puzzle and start looking inwards for the missing pieces that correspond to the missing pieces of skills and knowledge.

You start to realise how much there is for you to learn. For the first half of the year you learn lots of things, whereas somewhere in the middle you learn how to apply this knowledge. Some of you may have a crisis of confidence once you realise what is involved in terms of being a pharmacist, and the responsibilities and accountabilities that go with this. You may have learned these at university but it wouldn't have seemed as real then as it does now.

This period of time is usually when you start to consolidate what you know. When you come into a new rotation you have a fair idea of what to do and whom to ask. You are also at ease with the fact that you are starting again from the beginning, because your next supervisor has to reassess you to get an idea of your skills and abilities. You progress through the initial requirements fairly quickly because you have been through these before and know what to do. An example of this can be taking medication histories: you know what to do but have to prove to your supervisor that you can do this to his or her satisfaction.

You will have encountered many problems before but in the past you may have referred them to someone else; now you feel more able to tackle these problems yourself, safe in the knowledge that someone else is checking you and what you have done or said.

In the middle of the year you undergo your 26-week progress review at which your tutor informs you whether or not you are on the right track. If you are, this is the time to think about your role as a pre-reg. We often say to our pre-regs that the second half of the year is less about being a pre-reg and more about being a pharmacist, i.e. the pre-reg part of the title is now less important than the pharmacist part, bearing in mind that you are still not allowed to call yourself a pharmacist.

'Things started to fit together. Somehow, something is starting to click. At first, the rotations seemed to be all very different and didn't seem to have much to do with each other, but I realise now that in most rotations your goal is the same in that you make sure that things are safe for your patients. Although I am halfway through and things are starting to make sense, I'm also starting to think that I have so much more to learn and there is much more to being competent than I thought!'

As you approach the end of the training year, being a pharmacist is becoming a reality. This can be quite scary even if you thought that it would have been a fairly easy transition, mainly because you start to realise the responsibilities of being a pharmacist – your signature is going to count for something now.

In an ideal world, completing the pre-reg year and starting life as a professional pharmacist should be an easy transition; in many cases it is and you will feel no different to how you felt as a pre-reg. For others this transition can be quite traumatic because the safety net of someone checking your work has gone. You may find that you regress to what you were like when you started your pre-reg year, in that you start to doubt yourself and have to check the *BNF* (*British National Formulary*), check the *BNF* and then check it again, to make sure that the dose on the prescription is what it should be! This inevitably slows the process down and the staff around you may get frustrated with your slowness, but it is always better to get it right than to get it done quickly!

Depending on where you work after your pre-reg, your first few weeks can be very different. Some pre-regs take a short holiday before starting real work and others dive in as soon as they can.

'The closer it gets to the end, the more worried I am about being a pharmacist. At the beginning of the year I was very keen to be all signed off, but now I realise what a huge responsibility it is being a pharmacist and I'm starting to feel unprepared.'

TOP TIPS

- You may be a student at the start but should be a professional by the end
- Apply what you have learned at university
- Recognise your own strengths, weaknesses and gaps in skills and knowledge
- Be patient, listen to others and don't panic if you don't understand everything
- Develop your attitudes and behaviours to those of a pharmacist
- Put the patient in the centre of everything that you do
- People learn and develop at different rates so don't compare yourself too much with others

REFERENCE

Joint Formulary Committee. *British National Formulary*. London: British Medical Association and Royal Pharmaceutical Society of Great Britain, published six-monthly.

Section 2

A guide to rotations

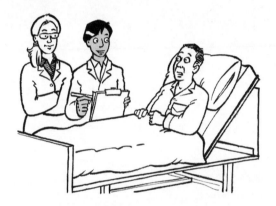

First rotation

6

You will feel a certain amount of trepidation when you start your first rotation, whichever area you may have been allocated to. You have just joined a new organisation and are still getting to grips with how things work and who all these people are. You are also unclear about other people's expectations of you as a pre-reg because you have never been in this position before. Your first rotation shows you very clearly how far you are from being a pharmacist, and this difference is uppermost in your supervisors' minds, as they probably have just had pre-regs who were at the end of their pre-reg training year and have now qualified. You should bear in mind that, for some supervisors, it can be very frustrating to train pre-regs from knowing nothing to practising competently, only for them to leave and the next lot of pre-regs to start from 'zero' again. This could mean that you are on the receiving end of some frustration from your supervisors, although it is not directed at you as an individual.

'I felt like we were thrown into the deep end. It was a steep learning curve. We did everything from first week. We were given a ward and had to do the ward ourselves. We dispensed from the satellite pharmacy, did stock top-ups, and did MI (medicines information) enquiries. In the first 2 weeks it was lots of pressure. It was hard but good. We had a taster of everything. I would wonder if other people cope under this pressure. We learnt so much in 6 weeks.'

'The majority of our work focused on technical aspects initially. Initially clinical knowledge was not being developed because we were taking lots time to do things. After a while the clinical side starts to develop as technical skills develop. It is good to acknowledge the technical side of the work to appreciate this. In terms of support from technicians and pharmacists, they expect a lot from you right from the beginning. Maybe they should have lower expectations if pre-regs are going there for their first rotation and provide orientation in the first week, with no unsupervised working in the first part of rotation.'

'My first rotation was on the wards, and I loved it – can't wait to go back. It's what I did my degree for, patient interaction – drug histories, counselling, picking up problems and making patients' lives better. At first I was apprehensive, thinking about how I am going to cope with it all. There was one patient with whom I found a problem and spoke to the doctor who changed the prescription. I knew that what I was saying was right but what is the boundary? I always would have passed it up because I am not a pharmacist yet. I thought that I must have done something wrong.'

'I've been in the dispensary for my first rotation and there are lots of processes to bring together. There are STILL lots of things to do. Initially, I felt like I was under people's feet. Felt like I was really helping in outpatients but in inpatients I felt like I needed a bit more reliance on other people in doing my job properly. It felt like a pressure cooker ....'

You may start your pre-reg training year with some degree of previous experience, which in some circumstances can put you at a slight advantage. But, whatever experiences you have had, you will still feel that you are starting from the beginning because each hospital has its own systems and standards. Even if you have done a summer placement at the hospital where you are now a pre-reg, you will feel that everyone's expectations of your work performance are different from those of a summer student.

Whatever rotation you start with, you will find that your supervisors assess your individual knowledge and skills before they are confident about letting you do anything unsupervised. At the start of your pre-registration training year, this undoubtedly happens every time that you work with a different pharmacist or technician. This could be very frustrating, especially when you are in a rotation, and your supervising pharmacists are themselves rotating so that, halfway through your rotation, you are working with an entirely new team of people who have not worked with you before, do not know what you are capable of and reassess you, making you feel as if you have to prove yourself again. Please tolerate this, because you must appreciate that your supervisors have to take responsibility for what you are doing under their supervision; in addition, be aware that, if anything goes wrong, you may also be liable.

'In my first rotation, I felt like people belittled the pre-regs. They stripped me down and made me humble. Initially nobody really cared. But after one rotation, I can already see a change in myself; I'm a lot calmer. If a situation arises, I think things through before doing. I used to just act on natural instincts and just go. I also used to be affected by others. But I have realised that this is not safe, so now I don't allow certain factors to get to me.'

Later in your pre-reg year, you will probably be 'tested' less, which means that people have certain expectations of your ability to do certain things. At this point, it is up to you to be honest with yourself, and with everyone else, about what you are, and are not, capable of.

It is useful to write some records of evidence from the beginning. This is a good way of recording your progression, and you'll be writing about very different issues throughout your training period. One way of looking at records of evidence is as a record of your CPD (continuing professional development), tracking your own learning and development, and reflecting on your own progress.

Another issue is how you show your supervisors, and ultimately your pre-reg tutor, that you are competent. In a community pharmacy, it is likely that you will work very closely with your pre-reg tutor, often side by side on a daily basis. This means that the community pharmacy tutor can directly observe what the pre-registration pharmacist is doing. In hospital pharmacy, your tutor probably won't work with you on a daily basis, because you are rotating around many different rotations, but you need to prove your competence to your tutor. This means that you must have some written evidence to prove that you have done the things that you say you have done. Your tutor will also rely on your supervisors' feedback and assessment in your different rotations, so you may well have appraisal meetings with each rotation to record what you have learned. In this way, your tutor can build up a picture of your developing practice and be sure that he or she is signing you off appropriately.

'The first rotation was interesting and quiet. I learnt a lot of stuff. It was a good base to start from. It was really the first time that I had met "real" pharmacists. I could see that their priority was their work, and that was interesting to see.'

'In my first rotation I went mad on the first day! I was given a folder and told to read. It was a hard day. It was only in the third week that I was able to process anything from beginning to end. When you don't understand the process you don't know when to ask for help.'

TOP TIPS

- Do not be scared if you have never been exposed to a particular rotation
- Be prepared to start from a zero baseline
- Learn the systems of work as soon as you can
- Be prepared to make mistakes
- If in doubt, ask
- Start writing good quality records of evidence

Ward-based pharmacy

7

Many people equate ward-based pharmacy with 'clinical' pharmacy, but we think that these are two very different things. In Chapter 2, we demonstrated our belief that all pharmacists, no matter where they are working, should regard themselves as 'clinical' pharmacists. Just because you are on a ward does not necessarily mean that you are thinking 'clinically'. It depends on your workplace what your ward duties are as a pre-reg, and in reality, when you start your ward based duties, many of these are of a technical rather than a clinical nature.

Ward-based pharmacy may include some of the following activities:

- Drug history taking or medicines reconciliation: this includes contacting GPs, speaking to patients and their carers, assessing patients' own medication, etc.
- Ordering of inpatient items for patients
- Checking ward stock, including controlled drugs and injectables
- Ward stock top-up
- Audit work
- Updating and maintaining ward folders
- Producing patient care plans
- Speaking to doctors, nurses and other ward staff to resolve any medicine-related problems
- Advising ward staff on correct administration of medicines, including injectable drugs
- Counselling patients or carers on their medication, e.g. device or warfarin counselling
- Contacting community pharmacists and GPs before patients are discharged to ensure smooth patient transfer back into the community
- Giving training sessions to ward staff on medicine-related issues
- Undertaking specific directorate work for specific teams of doctors; this may include financial, audit and formulary work
- Attending ward rounds

- Writing, screening and preparing discharge prescriptions
- Providing written patient reminders to aid patient compliance
- Providing answers to medicine-related enquiries for ward staff and patients.

Seeing or coming into contact with your first patient may be a daunting prospect, especially as you now have a job to do, as opposed to when you saw a patient on a ward as part of your undergraduate degree and the point of speaking to him or her was for your own learning.

The anxiety of interacting with patients is that you can never predict what they are going to say or do, and they might ask you a question to which you don't have the answer. If you are someone who needs to prepare before speaking to a patient, make sure that you do this. Bear in mind that you cannot prepare for every eventuality and at some point you will interact with patients who behave in a manner that you would not expect, or ask you questions for which you are unprepared.

When first encountering patients in the ward environment, always bear in mind that the people to whom you are talking may not be at their best – they are, after all, in hospital! So, if patients are not so willing to talk to you, do not take it personally – they may be tired or in pain.

Whenever you talk to patients, always introduce yourself clearly and state the reason why you are speaking to them. It can be confusing for patients to see many different healthcare professionals on the ward with little clue as to who is who and what they are all doing!

Talk to patients in plain English; avoid medical jargon such as 'I'm here to take your drug history' or 'I've come to prepare your TTO' (where a TTO is a discharge prescription) because this means little to patients and adds to their anxiety. A major role of pharmacy staff is translation of complex medical or pharmaceutical information into plain English that patients understand. You need to practise this type of communication until you get it right because it is hard to strike the right balance and not end up being condescending to a relatively knowledgeable patient.

For most interactions with patients, it is useful to ascertain their baseline knowledge and work from there. We always ask patients what the doctors have already told them, or what they already know, because this is a useful place to start.

'I felt like I was thrown in at deep end. For the first few days, I saw what my pharmacist did, then started to do drug histories myself. Then progressing with problems and making recommendations to doctors. I then went round each bed to see what I could spot for my pharmacist. Towards the end of the rotation, I could go up on my own and do drug histories and get information and I was itching for more. It is useful to learn that black and white becomes grey in certain patients.'

The ward environment is a great learning experience, not just from patients' notes and drug charts that you read. The other healthcare staff on the ward are a great source of information and learning too. It is interesting to speak to doctors, nurses and other healthcare professionals because it can be surprising how many different views of one patient different professionals have. Remember that different healthcare professionals have had extensive training in their particular field. so do not be afraid to ask them what the problems are from their points of view, in the same way as them not being afraid to ask pharmacy about drug-related issues.

One other source of learning is from the patients themselves, especially those with long-term conditions. There are many 'expert' patients out there. Always acknowledge patients' expertise in their own conditions and listen to their points of view, because they are the people who really know about their own condition and treatment – they are the ones with the condition after all.

When you first get up onto a ward, initially you won't know what to do, even if you have been given some clear instructions and there are clear expectations of your performance. The problem with the ward environment is that there are so many things going on that it is easy to be distracted and confused.

You have to recognise that you do not know everything; in fact, you probably feel like you don't know ANYTHING – in real life, not much matches the textbook learning that you were taught on your undergraduate course.

Your major source of information in the ward environment is your trusty *BNF* (*British National Formulary*). Many of the answers to many queries on the ward can be answered by referring to this text, but you will also quickly realise that not everything is contained within this text, and that you (under the supervision of your pharmacist) need to make decisions on what to **do** with the information found in the BNF. This type of decision-making requires some critical thinking on your part, which takes a while to develop. There are obviously limitations to the information inside the BNF; when this occurs you need to utilise the vast information resources in the hospital's medicines information department.

The major anxiety of ward work is that you cannot predict what people are going to ask you and you feel useless when you cannot solve somebody's problem or give ward staff a satisfactory answer. If you are somebody who likes to be prepared fully before embarking on anything, you will find working on the ward difficult at first because you can never predict what is going to happen on the ward. All you need to remember is that you must act within your competence at all times and refer everything else appropriately. If you are undertaking ward work towards the end of your pre-registration training year, and have had some prior experience of ward work, referring appropriately becomes more difficult to do, because you may be unsure what you are and are not competent in and you may not know the boundaries of your practice. At this point, you need to be careful not to overstep the mark, and act inappropriately without supervision from a pharmacist.

If you are rotating through different wards, and different specialities, you have to consider the fact that different wards have different systems of work, and do not presume that, if things work one way on one ward, the same applies to a different ward. Also, different pharmacists with whom you are working all work slightly differently. Don't let this confuse you; just learn from all the pharmacists around you and pick out the bits of practice that you think are great and incorporate them into your own practice.

You might feel anxious before going on to a ward if you think that you need to know lots of clinical 'stuff'. The reality of ward work is that anything you don't know you can look up. Ward work is not about what and how much knowledge you have, but about solving problems – about displaying critical thinking, always looking at everything in a critical manner and always asking 'why'. Another major issue is figuring out what to do first and which patient to see first. When you go up to a ward for the first time, it can be incredibly confusing and disorganised. With increasing time on the ward, you start to distinguish between things that need to be done urgently and things that can wait.

'It's complicated on the medical ward. Not black and white. I've learnt that the role of pharmacist on the ward is to question everything. You need to find the reason behind anything. You want to know why. Monitoring of patients on multiple drugs can be complicated. You need to be able to prioritise, knowing which patients are more important and why. You need to look at new patients – the whole picture of the patient. You have to sort out more complicated issues first. It is a challenge taking responsibility for what you are doing!'

'The surgical ward was really difficult to understand. Everyone had tubes down them, you don't learn that in uni. I felt like I learnt a lot. Learning which patients to see. They were all on loads of medicines and were old and complicated. I didn't really understand what to do. By the end I would see patients first that were on drugs like vancomycin, gentamicin, warfarin, etc. The two junior doctors on the ward did not know what they were doing. Every chart had something wrong with it. The nurses and doctors did not understand what a pre-reg was – so I kind of learnt to work around it. I would discuss problems with pharmacist X and then get back to people. It was really interesting. My major learning points were dealing with problems and thinking outside the box. Pharmacy has a big input on this type of ward. I felt that. The doctors would see me and call me over for pharmacy input. I felt really needed. By the end I knew the doctors and the nurses. Looking at drug charts – from not knowing what is wrong to thinking about what is the most important thing that is wrong. It's to do with your thought process.'

One of your major roles in the ward environment may be to take drug histories, or perform medicines reconciliation. This involves looking through lots of different sources to build up a picture of patients' medicine usage. You probably need to speak to the patient and to contact his or her GP. Contacting a GP may be a daunting task because you may fear that he or she may ask you questions to which you do not know the answer. Well, it is ok to say that you don't know! In addition, it is likely that you don't get through to the GP at first, but talk instead to the receptionist or other admin staff. Remember that many of these admin staff have not had any formal 'medical' training and may misread or misinterpret information on patients' records, so be sure to pitch your request for information to them correctly.

Every time that you go onto a ward with a different pharmacist, you will find that each has his or her own standards and lets you do things at different levels of supervision. As you are acting under a pharmacist's supervision, you can understand why they want to keep a close eye on you at first, to ensure that you are working to the expected standard. As a general rule, every time you work with a new pharmacist, you should expect him or her to supervise you more closely, and you may not be allowed to do many things without being directly supervised. As your supervising pharmacist becomes more familiar with the standard of your work, you will find that the level of trust in you increases and, by the end or a long rotation or towards the end of your pre-registration training, you may be expected to look after some patients as if they were your sole responsibility.

One of the best ways to solve the problem of constantly proving yourself is to show your records of evidence, where you have been signed off on particular activities, to your supervising pharmacist. Depending on how you have progressed during the year, you may have been signed off as competent for some performance standards (e.g. medication history) so you can show this to your supervisor to prove that you can actually do things.

The problem arises when there is no day-to-day continuity in the person looking after you. Every time that you work with somebody new, it is like starting from square one; this can be very frustrating, especially if you feel that you are working relatively independently. There are ways in which you can mitigate this to a certain degree, e.g. if you provide good written records such as logs or testimonials re. the level of your practice with other pharmacists, your new supervising pharmacist may take this into account. It is also useful to be very proactive in what you do. Never sit back and let your supervisor totally dictate what you can and cannot do. Throughout your training, you must always be at the forefront, pushing your own boundaries. After all, at the end of your pre-registration training, you will be expected to do all of these things competently, confidently and without supervision!

'There were similarities and differences with the pharmacists that I was with. Neither pharmacist X nor pharmacist Y got stressed, but they were not the same. Y was very methodical – had a checklist. X went on instinct – this was good but when will I get to be like that? Y knows her guidelines. X is using her experience. What they would pick out as important would be different. It was really useful to compare practice.'

Be aware that not all ward-based pharmacists are comfortable having pre-regs with them. Good clinical skills do not necessarily equate with good teaching skills. Some pharmacists have vast knowledge and expertise in certain clinical areas, and many years of experience in their chosen speciality, but they may have forgotten how they got there and not be able to communicate with a pre-reg at his or her level. Therefore they may assume that you know things that you can't do. It may even be that you have spent a few rotations in other areas such as dispensary, medicines information or technical services, and have not been to a ward before. There can be a tendency for pharmacists to compare you with a pre-reg who has just finished that rotation and can do much more than you.

'I most enjoyed taking drug histories and counselling. I least enjoyed contacting the prescriber because pharmacist Z made me feel stupid. I had conflict with Z. Z did not allow me to amend TTOs. The conflict made me feel stupid. I was going to cry. Z was stressed. After I knew that, it made me feel better. But I do not agree that Z should be doing things like that. I'm not going to be like Z. I was taught drug histories by Z – but he did not have to go through the whole list as I knew what I was doing! Z is very keen to teach but I do not like Z's style.'

Some pharmacists have a fantastic manner with patients and can communicate and get along well with both patients and staff; others do not. Although it is useful to see good practice that you can emulate and incorporate into your own practice, it can be argued that it is more valuable to see practice that you would regard as not being so good. It is useful to find practice with which you disagree and that makes you think about all the things that you WON'T do as a pharmacist!

Pharmacy technicians are increasingly being employed to work on wards as medicine management technicians. Their role on the wards may include taking drug histories, including contacting GPs, dispensing discharge prescriptions and ordering medicines for patients. As you may start with the more technical aspects of ward work, your roles may overlap significantly. The difference in your role as a pre-reg is that, when you have mastered the technical elements of ward-based pharmacy work, your role will extend beyond these technical jobs, so you have to start thinking about solving the problems that might be identified when a patient's drug history has been obtained. This is when your thinking changes from 'what' you are doing to 'why' you are doing it. Most medicine management pharmacy technicians have undergone a thorough training programme and are accredited to undertake certain tasks, which is what you will be doing as well, and in some hospitals you may find that you go through the same training using the same paperwork.

Obviously, your pharmacist will delegate work to you, but remember to keep an eye on what your pharmacist is doing. When you are the pharmacist, you will be doing all the things that your supervising pharmacist is doing, so what exactly is that?

How much you do on the ward depends on when your ward rotation falls within your training year, because you will find that many skills from other rotations are transferable to the ward environment; you will feel more capable of working in a ward environment towards the end of your training. Your supervising pharmacist will also realise this, and definitely capitalise on your skills if you have just done an extensive rotation in dispensary, for instance!

As a pre-reg, expect to be appropriately supervised when you are on a ward. Your hospital should have some rules about the definitions of supervised and unsupervised practice. But there could be times when you find that you are, momentarily, the only member of pharmacy staff on the ward. Don't panic! You can always find someone to refer to via a phone or a bleep. If you are expected to undertake some duties without a supervisor on the ward, it should have been clearly defined what you can and cannot do on the ward in these circumstances. Note that one of the performance standards is for you to be able to recognise your own limitations and refer appropriately, so there are opportunities for you to write more records of evidence.

Towards the end of the pre-reg training year, you may be expected to take on some duties as if you were acting as the pharmacist, e.g. you may be allocated a small cohort of patients for whom you are responsible. You will probably have to feed back what you have done to your supervising pharmacist so that he or she can check it. This increased responsibility of looking after your own patients is a real test of your abilities as a pharmacist and good practice for when you are qualified.

When on the wards, be careful to think about what your supervising pharmacist asks you to do. Think about the legal ramifications of what you do. There may be many things that hospital pharmacists do in the normal course of their daily work that may be considered illegal under the Medicines Act, but it is done commonly because it is accepted as custom and practice. For example, hospital pharmacists commonly endorse or change prescriptions on drug charts, such as substituting a formulary alternative of a drug for a non-formulary one. Be careful to distinguish this from legal requirements, because the law is what is examined in your registration exam at the end of your training, not what might be commonly practised in your hospital pharmacy department. There may be occasions when you need to refer to the *Medicines, Ethics and Practice* guide (RPSGB) to see what you can, or cannot, do, particularly in relation to controlled drugs.

'There were lots of guidelines in surgery. You try not to deviate into surgical procedures. Concentrate on things like pain control. What you can and can't take before surgery, antiemetics, laxatives, IG/IJ [intragastric/intrajejunal] guidelines. I didn't know what to expect at first. You don't have time to do everything so have to prioritise your workload, as you don't have time to see some patients. For instance some patients with no PMH who were previously fit and well with no meds. It's an important lesson to learn.'

'There are SO many patients, come in for lots different things – broad spectrum. Not all patients get equal attention – they are all so different. But you have to prioritise your patients – good for knowing which patients you should and don't need to see. You can't jeopardise the care of a more needy patient by seeing patients that don't need to be seen by you for the sake of "completeness". There's no time and no point to faff around.'

TOP TIPS

- Always distinguish between custom and practice and the law, because you will be examined on the law
- Develop some good relationships with the staff on the ward and you will find that your influence grows
- Never practise beyond your competence, because you risk patient safety
- 'Clinical' knowledge comes with practice, so never stop looking things up
- Write records of evidence to demonstrate your competence in a range of activities
- If you have been signed off for a performance standard, make sure that you show your pharmacist but continue to work at that standard

REFERENCES

Joint Formulary Committee. *British National Formulary*. London: British Medical Association and Royal Pharmaceutical Society of Great Britain, published six-monthly.

RPSGB. *Medicines, Ethics and Practice: A guide for pharmacists and pharmacy technicians*. London: Royal Pharmaceutical Society of Great Britain, published annually.

Patient services

8

'Patient services' is a term that is widely used to describe all the pharmacy services that are provided through the dispensary. For argument's sake, we define patient services as everything that happens in the dispensary, and stores, to effectively enable the patient to walk away with their medication.

Patient services cover all steps involved in screening, receiving, dispensing, supplying ward stock items, and final checking of all the medicines that are needed within the hospital, whether as inpatient items, stock items, controlled drug prescriptions or ward requisitions, trial drugs, unlicensed drugs, named patient drugs, discharge prescriptions, outpatient prescriptions, etc.

No matter where pharmacy is going to in the future, it is highly likely that a major pillar of pharmacy activity is through patient services. We say repeatedly to our pre-regs that the core skills of a pharmacist are dispensing and checking – it does not matter how much you think you know clinically, if the correct medicine is not supplied in the correct regimen with the correct instructions to the correct patient then the clinical part is useless! This is why so much importance is put on this at pre-registration trainee level, and why at least one whole section of the pre-reg performance standards has been dedicated to these activities – section C1, Managing the Dispensing Process – consisting of 12 performance standards, not to mention the many performance standards that dispensing and checking in the dispensary touch on outside these specific performance standards.

Types of prescriptions and orders seen in a hospital pharmacy department differ from those of a community pharmacy. There is a wider range of different documentation which at first is bewildering because the range of medicines encountered in a hospital dispensary can be vast, especially if your hospital offers many different specialisms.

In sharp contrast to a community pharmacist, there are many different types of prescriptions, requisitions and order forms with which you come into contact. For outpatient prescriptions there may be FP10s, A&E and outpatient prescriptions, and doctors' own prescriptions. For inpatient items there may be inpatient order forms, stock requisitions and discharge prescriptions, all of which have different formats. It takes a little while to figure out which form is for what purpose!

'Having had a lot of community experience, I can say that working in a hospital dispensary is very different. I had a preconceived idea that it was going to be similar to Boots but it's so different. It's busy but it's a good kind of pressure and I'm enjoying myself. I've completed my dispensing log and I'm getting there with my screening log. Done my CDs and am in the middle of doing my counselling log. I've learnt a lot. I'm actually looking at what the drug is and clinically screening – I've found out that it is very important to look at the drug. There's a lot more to it than I first thought!'

As well as handling the medicines available from the dispensary, you will probably also be handling patients' own medication, especially if you dispense and check discharge prescriptions. Remember that, no matter where the medicines have come from, all items need a stringent check to ensure that the right medicine has been prescribed to the right patient at the right regimen, and also that the quality and the physical state are of the highest quality.

Your first day in the dispensary will probably feel like a nightmare, especially if it has been a particularly busy day and there are lots of people rushing around with lots of things, and you asking what seem to be silly questions every few seconds! You will probably have an overwhelming sense of uselessness and of getting in everybody's way. Your usefulness will definitely improve when you slowly identify the systems at work in your hospital dispensary.

Hopefully you will have attended some kind of induction that enables you to feel vaguely oriented, and where some friendly and helpful faces have been identified.

'When I got into the dispensary I was raring to go. It can get busy! It was quite draining – it's hard when you don't know stupid things and can't find things. I had to keep asking what to do next. I realised that I needed to know the technical things. When it's busy you just have to get on and do what you can.'

At first, obviously you do not know where things are kept, but, as with any dispensary, there is a certain logic to how everything is laid out. It may help to follow a prescription from being received, all the way through to it being given to a patient, to understand the workflow in your dispensary. It may also be helpful to undertake some stock checks. Although you may think that this is dispensary staff getting a pre-reg to do a menial task, stock checks are useful in allowing you to get to know the layout in the dispensary, because it is not as simple as having drugs put in alphabetical generic name order. There may be many nooks and crannies where different types and sizes of products are kept, and the check also allows you to identify drugs that need refrigeration.

The layout of a hospital dispensary generally has the following rules:

- Drugs are in alphabetical order of generic name.
- Oversize items appear on any shelving that can contain that item.
- Any items that are not on the hospital formulary either appear in a separate section or are clearly labelled as non-formulary, clinical trial, etc. These should be housed with their associated paperwork nearby, because the record-keeping requirements of these items are stringent and need to be adhered to.
- Different formulations of drugs may have their own separate section, i.e. tablets and capsules, inhalers, drops, fluids, injections, dressings, etc.
- Controlled drugs are kept in a locked cupboard – or many cupboards in a dedicated controlled drugs room – ideally with a separate dispensing area where all the records are also kept.

If your hospital pharmacy dispensary has a dispensing robot, the main bulk of the dispensary stock is kept there. Note that the robot takes only unbroken original packs, so there may be additional shelving in the dispensary for keeping broken packs. The robot is basically an automated stock and picking system. Although there should be no picking errors when using a dispensing robot, errors can occur at a number of different stages involving humans.

'On my first day I thought "who is looking after me?". I just got on with it and dispensed some things. Asked random people what to do. It was a bit disjointed. I started all the log sheets all at once – no one was there to tell me what to do with them. My dispensing log was completed at the third attempt. What sort of errors did I make? Stuff like eyedrop bottles with labels on the wrong way round – that was because I had not had my morning break. I was really annoyed and depressed at having to restart my log at 180 items. You've got to accept that errors happen but you have to think about why it happened.'

Your first few days of dispensary work will make you very tired – especially your feet! This is why dispensary staff place great importance on tea breaks; if you are working hard in the dispensary, you definitely need to take all your allocated breaks. Be sure to take them on time too, because you may delay other people's breaks if you are late going on yours – and people do not thank you for this.

At first, you will be asked to perform the more technical aspects of dispensing. This allows you to get used to the process of dispensing drugs, and the steps that need to be completed correctly. In the beginning you will probably struggle with the most basic of tasks, such as where to physically stick the label on the medicine container. The first time that you are asked to produce a label on the computer system may also cause you some stress and you won't have a clue as to how the labelling system works, let alone think about short codes!

Remember that a range of dispensary staff operate in the dispensary, not just pharmacists, and that each staff member has an important role to play within the dispensary. Do not be surprised if the person in charge of the dispensary is not a pharmacist. These days, it is highly likely that the dispensary manager is a technician. Whether the dispensary manager is a pharmacist or a technician is not important. What IS important is that this person is the one in charge and so you should be directed by him or her in the work that you do.

There will be many different policies, procedures systems that you need to follow while in the dispensary, and at first what you need to do is confusing. There are many, many folders filled with standard operating procedures that you need to follow, and different pieces of paper that need to be filled in depending on whether the dispensed medicine is on the hospital formulary, non-formulary, unlicensed, part of a clinical trial or a specially manufactured item. It takes time to untangle all the requirements that working in a busy hospital demands, but don't worry, with practice and your familiarisation with how the systems work, things eventually become clear and you don't feel stupid having to ask somebody what to do next a million times a day.

You may find that, when the dispensary is busy, you are called in from other rotations to help. Although this may be perfectly reasonable, you should question why the dispensary takes precedence over other areas, especially if you may be the only member of staff holding the fort in your particular rotation. The dispensary is undoubtedly important, but the work that you are doing in another section is equally important, and you have to weigh up whether or not you can be spared to go into the dispensary. Remember that you, as the pre-reg, have the obligation to learn about all the different sections of your pharmacy department and you need to become competent in all of these areas, not just the dispensary.

As part of your dispensary training you are required to dispense, label, screen and check a certain number of items before dispensary staff deem that you can do any of these processes correctly. You will be given paperwork to fill in as evidence that you have achieved your set goals. As there are multiple points in the dispensing process where errors can be picked up, it is hoped that any errors that you make will be identified and rectified before the item leaves the dispensary. These errors are massive learning points, because they may expose areas of your dispensing and checking process that need to be more systematic. It is useful at first to devise and write down a self-checking procedure and adhere to this. Every member of pharmacy staff has their own internal checklist that they go through; it does not matter in what order you check your work, only that, at the end, everything that needs to be checked has been covered. You will find that most dispensaries have some logs or paperwork for you to complete that is based on the paperwork for accredited checking technicians (ACTs). ACTs undergo a thorough training programme before they are allowed to check prescriptions that they have not dispensed, and have to be regularly revalidated by passing a dispensary test. On most occasions, once you have completed your pre-reg training, you may never be assessed, or revalidated, again for your dispensing – in your whole career!

It is likely, however, that you will make mistakes. Although experienced pharmacy staff are generally able to bear the responsibility of what they are doing and therefore accept the fact that they make errors every now and again, the first error that you make may come with some emotion, especially if a patient has subsequently taken the wrong medication as a result of your error.

'I couldn't believe it when I found out that I had dispensed that antibiotic for the patient when the allergy was clearly stated; I felt so bad, like I was responsible for the error even though the pharmacist checking it was responsible. I had a bit of a cry and then spoke to the pharmacist who explained that these things happen and the patient didn't actually take the antibiotic and had brought it back.'

The first time that you have to query a prescription with a doctor will be a daunting one, especially if you are working on outpatients and the patient is waiting patiently for the medication. The stress comes from not knowing how the doctor will respond to your request and also how assertive you can be, especially if you feel that you do not have the whole picture of the patient's condition. Although you can never totally predict what will happen, you CAN be prepared for the interaction by thinking through what the doctor might subsequently ask you. For example, if you are going to speak to the doctor to say that you cannot provide a particular medicine for whatever reason, it would not be unreasonable for the doctor to then ask 'what alternative do you suggest?' – so it would obviously be wise to think of this before even picking up the phone.

'I was calling a doctor to change the antibiotic on the prescription because the patient had said he was allergic to penicillin and had the BNF out on the right page, I was really nervous because everyone had said that he was not a nice doctor. When I started talking to him he was really nice and thanked me for calling him back but then he asked what alternatives we kept in the pharmacy.... I hadn't thought of that and was going to recommend that he prescribe X, I had to say that I would find out and call him back. When I called him back, he was obviously in the middle of something because he was short with me and said that he would write the prescription if I could ask the patient to come back and see him. I was going to say that I could change the prescription for him but he had put the phone down; I had to go and explain to the patient who was not happy.'

You will find that sometimes you make some clinical judgements with limited information available to you. When you are in a ward environment, it can be easier to make judgements about whether or not something is appropriate; it may not be so easy to find this information if all you have in front of you in the dispensary environment is a piece of paper with a few words on it and no context. Life in the dispensary teaches you with what minimum amounts of information you will be comfortable when making a decision.

The dispensary could be an environment where a lot of conflict happens. Although this may be an uncomfortable prospect for you, view it as a good opportunity to demonstrate your ability to deal with conflict appropriately – which happens to be one of the performance standards! As many of your encounters with medical and nursing staff are via the phone, there is much more opportunity for misunderstanding to take place; this teaches you good communication skills too! Patients may also cause conflict; just bear in mind that some patients may have waited for several hours to be seen by several different types of healthcare staff and they baulk when faced with another hour's wait for their prescription! Sometimes pharmacy gets it in the neck purely because, for many patients, it is the last stage of a hospital visit filled with many delays and waits!

With a bit of dispensing practice under your belt, you may find that different checkers – be they pharmacists or accredited checking technicians – require slightly different standards from you. Although there is obviously a minimum standard as required by law, most checkers operate at a much higher standard than this, and, although what you have dispensed may be sufficient by law, the person who is checking your work at that moment may require more, and each individual checker has slightly different standards, or particular standards for particular types of prescriptions. Dispensing a prescription in a particular way for one checker may not mean that another checker does not return the prescription to you to be re-dispensed. Although this may be frustrating, you will understand when you develop your own standards and requirements from other dispensers.

The end point for any dispensary training is to be able to practise at a dispensary level with as few errors as possible (preferably no errors obviously!). As mentioned previously, dispensing and checking are the core skills of a pharmacist; if you cannot get these two things right, you cannot be a pharmacist and none of the other skills matters.

Most hospital programmes have pre-regs who work in several dispensary rotations, often in different dispensaries and sometimes on different sites. The advantages are that this allows you to work with different systems and different people because the layout of every dispensary is different. The downside can be that you need to ensure that you have good records of what you have done, what you need to do and what you have been signed off for. This means that you can continually progress from the technical aspects of dispensing at the start to the clinical aspects of the prescriptions by the end (hopefully!)

'Six weeks of dispensary changed the way I dispensed. On receiving prescriptions, I realised that taking histories is important. On inpatient dispensing I didn't just do dispensing, I screened the prescriptions while I dispensed. You check every single drug. You don't have to be told to do this. The focus was on what is happening with these prescriptions. Prescriptions are like puzzles; you use lots of information to put things together and make sure everything fits.'

'I had no previous dispensary experience before starting my rotation. It was definitely a steep learning curve. I felt like I made a lot of progress. When I started my dispensing log, I made two minor errors, then there was a spelling error on someone else's label so made three minor errors and I had to start my dispensing log all over again. It made me realise that I should be dispensing from the prescription and not from a label that someone else has produced.'

'I had two blocks of dispensary with my clinical rotation sandwiched in between. I didn't realise how much I had to do in dispensary! When I came back for my second dispensary block, I felt a lot more efficient, more focused. It hit home that I was not going back to dispensary. Screening TTOs became easier in the second dispensary block because the process is exactly the same as on ward.'

'When I first started dispensary I was scared. I didn't know what I was doing and how things worked. I was getting sick of myself asking things. I started in inpatients. I had had dispensary experience in Boots. Uni pharmacy practice lessons did not help much. In my dispensing log I made one error – an incorrect quantity on the label. Did one log at a time. Sometimes I ended up dispensing even when I should have been concentrating on screening some prescriptions – it's so busy so you don't know if you'll be useful. If you try to screen, you are so slow and you feel like you're getting in the way.'

Pre-regs all encounter working in stores in some way or another. In some hospitals you may be required to undertake 'top-ups'; this is where you go to a ward and take a stock check of what medicines are on the ward and what needs ordering. You then complete an order sheet to go to stores for the medicines to be picked up and distributed to the wards; you may even be asked to do the picking and packing into ward boxes. This activity is generally undertaken by pharmacy support staff but, thinking about it, it is one of the most critical aspects of getting medicines to the wards. Some experience of seeing how this process works, and what problems may occur, is vital for you to understand why medicines are not on the ward when you expect them to be. They don't appear there just by magic!

Many pre-regs complain that they do not consider this good use of their time because 'I did not spend 4 years at university to come here and pack boxes'. We recommend that you think about this activity in a different way, from a risk and governance point of view:

- Where are the risks in the system that may result in wrong medicines being sent to the ward?
- What is the process for informing ward pharmacy staff that medicines are out of stock and have not been sent to the ward?
- What is the process for informing the nurses on the wards?
- If a medicine is out of stock, who makes the decision to provide an alternative? If so, what does he or she base the decision on?
- On the ward, what risks are there in terms of picking errors by the nurses?

- Are medicines stored alphabetically or is there another system? If there is another system, do you understand it? If not, what is the risk of a nurse not understanding it either?
- Are look-alike and sound-alike medicines kept near each other?
- What happens if generic medicines are in the ward cupboards and they are different brands with different packaging? What are the risks?
- Are high-risk medicines such as penicillin-containing antibiotics and certain injections kept separately from other medicines?
- How is stock on the ward rotated to ensure that no out-of-date medicines are on the ward?

The above are just some of the things that you need to think about. The NHS takes risk management very seriously and organisations such as the National Patient Safety Agency (NPSA) provide national guidance on some high-risk medicines in terms of their safe storage and administration.

TOP TIPS

- Always think critically about prescriptions – never just blindly follow a process without asking 'why?'
- Don't be afraid of making an error – finding the boundaries of your practice can teach you a lot about yourself
- When you do make an error, think whether there was something that you could have done to prevent it from occurring
- If you find that you are losing concentration and are not focused on your work, take a break; errors often occur near break times and at the end of the day when you are rushing and not concentrating
- Make sure that you keep good records of your progress through patient services so that you can keep track of what you need to do throughout the year
- What are the risks to patient safety when considering safe storage of medicines on the wards?

Medicines information

'Medicines information is not really my thing.'
'There is too much reading to do in medicines information.'

These are just some of the comments that pre-regs often make about medicines information (MI). This could not be further from the truth because MI is a fundamental part of hospital pharmacy; it is just that some people do not perceive it to be as sexy as other rotations. We often find, as you will as well, that there is a love–hate relationship for pre-regs in the MI rotation – either they love it or they hate it, there tends to be no middle ground – the 'Marmite effect' as we term it! Even those pre-regs who hate the MI rotation realise the benefits and the transferable skills that they gain from MI. For those of you who may not have an MI rotation, or indeed an MI centre, most of the skills and knowledge are gained in different ways – you just won't realise it! When you ask questions, on the phone or in person, you are effectively using a questioning strategy to find out as much as you can about the problem and similarly, when trying to answer a question, or query, you follow a systematic approach. A Google search takes you only so far!

This chapter focuses on a typical pre-reg rotation in MI. Whether it is a large MI centre or a desk and a phone tucked away in someone's office, the learning and issues are quite similar.

THE FIRST FEW DAYS

Depending on which rotation you have just come from, the first few days in MI can be very different to what you have been used to. If you have just finished a rotation in the dispensary or on the wards, you are used to a very busy working environment where you are always on your toes and all your deadlines seem to be immediate. It is quite easy to quantify what you have been doing. MI is just not like that; it can be very busy with important deadlines but when the MI team get busy you find that they become quieter and go into their shells as they concentrate on the work at hand. This is the exact opposite of what happens elsewhere and it may come as a culture shock to some of you.

'MI was like watching paint dry. It's not me. I can't sit somewhere in silence and read. I was falling asleep. The workbook was mind numbing. When I was actually answering enquiries, it felt good actually doing some work. I learnt some things that I will not forget now. I don't think I really like long enquiries. I wouldn't like to have an MI job – this is good because at least I know now. It IS good to know where to look for information. Now I know that I need more information than is volunteered with queries.'

There are many different types of MI rotations and centres. In the smaller hospitals there may not even be an MI centre, just a desk with a phone and a bookshelf with books and resources. The MI pharmacist may well have other responsibilities and not always be at the MI desk. There may be an answer-phone service for MI enquiries that are non-urgent directing the caller to their ward-based or clinical pharmacist for patient-related enquiries. The other extreme is a regional MI centre that is staffed by many pharmacists and pharmacy technicians, and is very well resourced with all the latest databases and access to a wide variety of online resources. In a larger centre you may be introduced to all the staff at the start of the rotation but may never speak to some of them because their roles and responsibilities are not related to the enquiry. When you start your rotation in MI it is important for you to find out the team structure and to whom you have to report.

Lots of things can go on in a large MI centre, including managing the hospital formulary, providing clinical governance support for medicine management, writing supporting documents for drugs and therapeutics committees, or horizon scanning for new, or potentially new, medicines that are in clinical studies. This list is not exhaustive and you may find that your MI centre does some or all of these.

The bread-and-butter activity of all MI centres is answering enquiries from hospital-based healthcare professionals as well as from the general public. This is where most of your training time will be spent because answering an enquiry remains a fundamental skill for all pharmacists. There are minimum standards for all MI centres, provided by the national MI group, United Kingdom Medicines Information (UKMI). First you will be asked to go through an MI training pack because this is standardised nationally and all pre-regs are required to undertake similar training packs, or workbooks. This requires you to read through various chapters that guide you through how to answer an enquiry and, perhaps more importantly, how to ask the right questions at the right time in the right order. Good questioning techniques mean that you can get more of an overview of the problem and therefore be in a much better position to answer the question. This is the activity that most pre-regs find a bit boring, to be frank, because they have been used to rushing around in the dispensary and on the wards and see other pharmacists answer questions all of the time without necessarily having a structured approach to doing so. Paying particular attention to the activities in the workbook is an investment in your time because, when you do start getting your own enquiries, you will be practised at asking the right questions.

'I am worried with the amount of reading so I don't really enjoy it. I am indifferent. I have learnt how to communicate better with other healthcare professionals and patients. You need to tailor your answer and speak in appropriate language. You develop listening skills, researching and using resources properly. There are so many books that I didn't know existed, now I know where to look and I now know how to do it. I have learnt quite a lot. But sitting in a room looking at a computer is hard – I can't physically sit there all day.'

ANSWERING ENQUIRIES

Once you have read through the workbook and your supervisor has agreed that you can start answering enquiries, you start with some easy, straightforward enquiries. This is another of the frustrating stages for some of you. You may think that you already know the answer, so why go through all the reference texts? There are many reasons for this but from the point of view of your training it is to embed in your practice the structured approach to answering enquiries. As you start answering more complex enquiries, you may never reach one conclusive answer; when going through the different resources, you may find that the answer is becoming more unclear because the resources provide conflicting answers. A good example of this is when attempting to answer enquires relating to drugs in pregnancy because the use of a particular drug is often a risk–benefit decision taken by the prescriber, and your role is to provide the information for the decision to be made rather than make the decision yourself.

One thing that you may learn in MI is that the question first asked is not always the question in the mind of the enquirer. Examples of this are when a doctor asks what the dose of a specific medicine is or when a nurse asks how to administer a medicine. What they should really be asking is whether to prescribe or administer this medicine in the first place. As you get more experience with both answering enquiries and building your knowledge base of medicines, you can start to recognise medicines not routinely used in particular clinical areas which may raise alarm bells in your thinking – at least we hope that this will be the case.

As you become more practised at answering enquiries, your supervisor may start letting you answer the phone. All MI centres differ as to when they allow pre-regs to start answering the phone; sometimes this is early on in your rotation and other times later on. This depends on how you progress, as well as how much support you have. We have experience of some pre-regs who have been absolutely petrified of answering the phone in MI; they did not experience any difficulty in answering the phone in the dispensary or on the wards, but when in MI a ringing phone raised fears. On investigation this was because the pre-reg was scared that it might be a senior doctor on the phone and they wouldn't know what to say. One of the first things that you are taught is to take the details of the enquirer and as much detail as possible about the patient, if there is one. This is so that, if any other problems come to light, the enquirer can easily be contacted. A busy healthcare professional is not aware of the processes involved in answering an enquiry and how robust your search processes need to be, even for simple enquiries, so they inevitably want an answer straightaway. It is easy to imagine a nurse ringing the MI centre to ask how a particular medicine should be given with the phone under her or his chin and the injection primed and ready to be administered. It is critical that what you say is correct even if the nurse has to wait for the medicine to be administered.

Another thing that some pre-regs have commented on is that they do not know which questions to ask because they have never heard of the drug or the disease before and therefore have no idea where to start; although they have done the training in the workbook, they are worried that they may ask a completely inappropriate question and not understand the answer. This is where the support of the MI pharmacist becomes invaluable because there is no reason why you cannot refer the caller to the other pharmacist if you feel out of your depth. Remember to have all the details that you can about the enquiry before passing it on; if you do not know the drug or disease, ask the caller to spell it out to you and double-check the spelling with them – at which point it would be prudent to explain to them that you are a pre-reg and in training. Do remember that some letters sound different over the phone (S can be an F, P can be a B or a T, T can be a D, etc.).

'I thought it was going to be difficult. Answering phone calls when everyone is listening is a bit nerve wracking. From one week to the next week I've learnt a lot. I covered a range of subjects in enquiries. The skills that I've learnt are to be more confident over phone to healthcare professionals. I can now use resources. I'm getting used to being in a working environment and how to get on with people that you don't like.'

'I like MI a lot. All I do is chat all day. The MI workbook was done in 3 days. I'm not afraid of the phone. I'm more confident over the phone. It is nice that in MI "I am allowed to not know". Looking up stuff is totally within my comfort zone.'

Examples of other types of enquiry that may be encountered include identifying tablets and capsules. Some MI centres have databases for this; other centres would refer these enquiries to the regional MI centre. You will learn the questions that you need to ask to increase your chances of successfully identifying the tablet/capsule. The trick is to ask some clinical question in terms of what the medicine might be used for, as well as technical questions in terms of shape, colour and dimensions of the tablet/capsule.

LAW AND ETHICS

It may surprise some of you to learn that a lot of what you do in MI is challenging the law and making ethical decisions – not in the same way as in the dispensary, but you could need a reasoned approach when informing the enquirer of an answer, especially if the enquirer is a member of the public. You may not know if the enquiry relates to that person or someone he or she knows, or if any medicine is yet to be taken or has been taken. This is particularly so when dealing with enquiries about side effects or adverse drug reactions. It has been known for enquirers to ask such questions without providing the full reasons of why they are asking and who they are; sometimes they are concerned parents or relatives, or even journalists or members of the legal profession. How you tackle these enquiries is very different to the ones that you usually encounter in the hospital and you need to refer these to more senior colleagues for help and guidance. It is always worth finding out how they would approach such situations because, in a year or so, it may well be you who is faced with such a dilemma.

'MI was my biggest area of development in terms of knowing what questions to ask, trying to pre-empt what might be asked next, plus any extra advice. Sometimes there is no answer or there could be several answers. It's up to the person who enquired to make the clinical decision based on evidence. If there is conflicting information, you need to give a balanced answer and show both sides.'

The main challenge arises when you have to formally correspond with the enquirer in the form of a letter or an email. You need to be careful how you phrase some of the terms and not to lead the enquirer into an answer but to present the facts as they are. It is not up to you to make a decision but to provide the information for the enquirer to put into context and then make a decision. Unlike on the wards or in the dispensary, you may never find out what the outcome was and whether your information was useful. This depends on the nature of the enquiry and who was asking. As MI is a specialist service, whatever you write may be taken as gospel and, even if your name is at the end of the letter, you still represent pharmacy MI. This is why there are such strict standards for MI pharmacists when corresponding, because the written word is more permanent than the oral one.

As you can see from the pre-reg quotes below, this rotation is not everyone's cup of tea and the quotes show the range of experiences for pre-regs, together with the realisation that they all learned transferable skills in terms of answering queries.

'I really enjoyed MI. It was really good structure training. It was brilliant; I had such a good time. I really enjoyed myself. At first I was quite nervous and cautious before getting to know a situation. I worked through the UKMI book so had good background. Sometimes there is no black and white, no definitive answer – i.e. pregnancy queries – you need to weigh up risks and benefits. You need to tailor your answers to who you are giving the answers to – to make sure you don't scare the patient while still making them aware of risks.'

'I learnt how to use resources, i.e. drug use in pregnancy. I learnt how to speak on the phone. I learnt some transferable skills like the fact that it is best not to give an opinion, but to just state the evidence. It makes you be more careful about the advice and opinions that you might give in community. Opinions come with experience.'

'I really hated it to start with – don't like it as a rotation. I hate sitting at a desk all day, I have to be busy. I didn't really start doing things until 4 weeks. But now I have learnt SO much from it. MI teaches you how to be methodical, how to use resources, etc.'

'MI was my favourite rotation. You learn some very useful skills that are transferable, like learning how to write letters without using medical jargon. Phone answering was a bit scary at first but I improved. Everything is grey. You do everything in lots of depth, it is very clinical.'

'I did not know what to expect. The first 2 weeks I worked through the workbook. There was gradual increase in responsibility/confidence. I did a good range of enquiries. Initially MI did not come naturally. By the end it was wicked. I learnt so much stuff. You really get into the subjects that you are doing the enquiry in. I have also learnt that the BNF does not have all the information in it!'

'I learnt lots of things from looking at lots of resources. I need to remember these. I need to be methodical and to go through sources systematically. I've learnt that the information has to match the summary. You have to be direct due to legal issues and to document everything. Since you often don't have all the patient information, your information needs to be very structured and specific. You need to think about consequences of the information that you are providing. You cannot be prejudiced, as you get queries from patients from all backgrounds and cultures.'

'MI is not for me. I started answering the phone just recently. I repeated the information back to enquirer to ensure I got everything down. I don't like grey answers; I like yes or no. I have difficulty summarising information and writing letters. It takes a long time. If there is no right or wrong answer, you need to be sure about what you're writing.'

'I loved MI. I organised and prioritised queries. MI is good for problem solving. It is the only rotation where I felt I gained some responsibility. You take charge of your own queries, so there is massive satisfaction from my own workload. I had some weird enquiries where you think there's a clear-cut conclusion, but get contradictory information from different resources. So you need to make a judgement and interpret the information. You also need to think why that question is being asked.'

'MI was my favourite rotation. It felt tedious in the beginning though. But I liked that you are given responsibility and that you manage your own work-load. You can choose what you want to do and have the autonomy of working on your own workload. I felt responsible enough to handle things on my own. My biggest development was in confidence in dealing with different healthcare professionals and patients. You have to phrase things very differently to target your information. Answering the telephone was ok. I was scared at the beginning but knew I had to do it. I got less scared as the rotation went on. By the end of rotation, I loved it. How will this inform my clinical practice? MI changes your thought process. You know where to look for answers. I am more confident in giving answers to enquiries. I have learnt that you should have your facts straight and not to blag. Most enquiries in MI are more complicated than ones that might get asked in other areas. Documentation needs to be done because it is the procedure. A lot of things in medicines are hardly ever black and white. I'm always looking for that grey area – I like to see that there were shades are grey. Nothing's ever clear cut.'

TOP TIPS

- Be prepared to go through and read the training manual
- Adopt a logical and structured approach to enquiry answering
- Don't be scared of the phone
- Listen to the enquirer carefully and get their name and number
- Realise that there may never be a conclusive answer
- Note that your role is to provide information, not necessarily to answer the question
- Remember your law and ethics
- Use the same questioning and answering skills in other rotations

Technical services 10

Technical services is an over-arching rotation which can include a variety of different areas:

- Sterile manufacture (total parenteral nutrition [TPN], central intra-venous additive service [CIVAS] and chemotherapy)
- Non-sterile manufacture (extemporaneous preparation and bulk manufacture)
- Quality assurance/quality control.

We have to start by recognising that some pharmacy departments have made a decision not to offer the whole range of technical services available to them in the pre-reg year on a similar basis to not all clinical specialities being included in the pre-registration year. Having said that, technical services remain a fundamental aspect of hospital pharmacy and the skills gained from this rotation are transferable to the other rotations; experience in technical services may also be relevant for a career in the pharmaceutical industry. Some hospitals have links with other hospitals where you can go and undertake this rotation. If this is not the case you will probably have the opportunity to learn about technical services through teaching sessions with expert technical services staff or by visiting the units. It is unlikely that you will receive absolutely no input about this area in your training year.

Many pre-regs approach this rotation with some concerns because they do not know what to expect and think that they will find the rotation boring. They are usually pleasantly surprised at the end of the rotation and say that they did not expect it to be as interesting as it was. This comment may be because the rotation is not clinical and the work is not necessarily clinically focused, so you would not be seeing patients as an everyday part of your practice. In fact you may go through the whole rotation and not see a single patient.

STERILE AND NON-STERILE PRODUCTS

Some of you may have some experience of making sterile products from university, when working in a mock sterile unit, and certainly in lectures when you learnt about such things as methods of sterilisation. In technical services, you see some of these methods in real-life practice as well under-standing how, in a controlled environment, aseptic technique is fundamental to producing sterile products; compare this with what you may see in clinical areas where injectable medicines are prepared. The pharmacist takes accountability of all aspects of the production of aseptic products but does not necessarily get involved in their direct manufacture. Paperwork or, more correctly, documentation forms an important part of technical services. There is paperwork for everything – even how to wash your hands!

So what is the role of a technical services pharmacist and what do you learn from this rotation? One of the first things to which you are exposed is the numerous standard operating procedures that you need to go through and sign up to before you can put your hand to anything. Many pre-regs have said that this is the most boring part which means that the rotation can often start on the wrong foot. Don't worry, however, because, although the first few days can feel as if all you are doing is reading procedure after procedure, you are actually familiarising yourself with the working of the unit in terms of regulatory requirements. You learn that, for licensed manufacturing units, the Medicines and Healthcare products Regulatory Authority (MHRA) has a big role to play in terms of ensuring that work carried out in the unit con-forms to the regulatory requirements. Other regulatory bodies have a role to play, such as the Health and Safety Executive (HSE) and, of course, the Royal Pharmaceutical Society of Great Britain (RPSGB). You learn about the law, particularly the Medicines Act and how this is applied in this environment, rather than within community or hospital practice as you may have learned at university; you also learn about Section 10 of the Medicines Act and how unlicensed medicines are prepared.

As well as learning about the law, you learn about the design of a clean room, which involves learning about how clean rooms are graded in terms of cleanliness and sterility. There are different requirements for the cleaning and maintenance of clean rooms depending on their grade. You learn the differ-ences between an isolator and a laminar airflow bench, and what products are made in each. You definitely learn about environmental monitoring, which may seem a bit boring at the time; if you look at the bigger picture, however, you will understand the critical nature of this activity. Environmental moni-toring includes measuring airflows through inlet and outlet fans and particu-late matter coming out of an air filter (e.g. a HEPA filter – high efficiency particulate air filter), as well as monitoring of air pressures between positive and negative pressure rooms such as a clean room. All of this is critical because, if anything is not within allowed tolerances, work carried out in the unit may not be of the required sterility. Settle plates are usually used to identify external contaminants and if there any bacteria present that should not be. It can often be the role of the pre-reg to go into a unit and place settle plates in different areas and, once a particular batch of products is made, to remove these plates and send them off to quality control.

'I didn't really understand why we needed to do all of this monitoring until one day the filters became blocked and there was a mad panic to see if we could still use the unit; it made me realise why environmental monitoring was important because I was asked to report on what the readings were for the week leading up to today.'

'The other day the temperature in the unit became very hot; I know it's summer but the air conditioning unit must have been down. We had to shorten the expiry dates of some of the products and I was asked to look into their stability to see which ones would be affected. The other thing I learned was that on hot days you have to think about the people making the products because it can be hard for them to concentrate ... we ran short shifts for the technicians so that they could have lots of short breaks.'

As you will be one small part of a bigger process, or set of processes, it is important for you to understand where you fit in. Make the time to learn about the bigger picture in terms of why you are doing things in a certain way and why the legislation is the way that it is.

Let's start with the biggest bugbear of pre-regs – documentation. Why is this so important? If you are working in a licensed unit, the MHRA needs to know how safe the working systems are; they can only do this by reviewing the standard operating procedures, who has read and understood them, and how they have been modified in the wake of errors. The aim is to provide the safest possible system. Think about the types of patients who receive medications that are made in a sterile unit; it won't be patients who are well enough to take oral medications but those who are critically unwell and therefore the most vulnerable.

'On my first day I was given some massive files to go through and read SOPs [Standard Operating Procedures]; this was really boring and I could hardly keep my eyes open. I had just finished a rotation on the wards where I was rushing around and found it hard going sitting there all day reading SOP after SOP.'

Documentation allows managers of the unit to track how work systems have evolved over a period of time. An example of where a deficiency, the technical word for a problem, has occurred is when a pre-reg, involved with inputting a handwritten prescription to the computerised labelling system using a Windows-based programme with drop-down lists, picked the wrong strength of one of the ingredients. The lack of experience of this pre-reg meant that he did not realise that this was a mistake and the computer worked out a volume of ingredient based on an incorrect, weaker strength. When it came to selecting the ingredients to make the products, in this case a bag of TPN for a neonate, the usual, higher-strength ingredient was added to the tray and the batch number and expiry duly recorded. The person who checked this step of the process signed to say that the batch number and expiry date were recorded correctly but overlooked the wrong strength of the ingredient because that weaker strength was not routinely kept in the unit. The high volume was noted but not acted upon because the previous batch had been for adult TPN where the volumes are obviously higher. In the end, the error was spotted by the pharmacy technician actually making the product, and the correct worksheet was produced. This led to an investigation of how the process had produced the error and corrective action was taken.

The pre-reg involved was obviously upset and we talked about how the error could have occurred and how the work system could have been improved. The pre-reg was then able to input into how he made the mistake and offered suggestions to prevent this from happening. That was supposed to be that, but imagine our surprise when a year later another pre-reg reported doing exactly the same thing! On this occasion the error occurred for a different reason but changing the work system had resulted in a different set of risks. This shows how important pre-regs can be to the workings of the unit because they read an SOP (standard operating procedure) and follow it literally to the letter. It is critical that an SOP has no ambiguity in it and who better to test this than a pre-reg with little or no prior experience?

The other types of documentation are the following:

- Specifications, e.g. chemical raw materials, packaging materials and products that we make ourselves
- Manufacturing instructions (materials needed, quantities required and equipment used)
- Packaging instructions (the type and number of packaging and any specific packaging requirements).

It is up to you to learn what these are for and when they are used. You may find that your unit has a number of master documents that must be used each time that a product is made.

It is often said that working in technical services is very much like cooking. Have a look at any cookery book – there is a list of ingredients, the specifications, how much you need of each, what equipment you may need to make the product, the manufacturing instructions, and finally what to put your 'final product' in and how to store it – the packaging instructions. Easy really, except that any deviation from the instructions means that your final product may not be what it should be. Anyone who has experimented with cooking will tell you that sometimes things go wrong! This risk cannot be taken for granted when making medicines for critically ill patients, so you can now see why documentation is so important.

'I was sieving some powder to make tablets and because this was really boring I was thinking about the job interview I had that morning, what I answered well and what I did badly, when I realised that I had forgotten to put the collecting tray under the sieve. I saw it on the bench and wondered what it was doing there but did not think anything of it at the time; then I saw the pile of powder on the floor and didn't know whether to laugh or cry. The boss then came in and was really angry at my stupidity. The amount of paperwork I had to do to explain why a batch of tablets could not be made was unbelievable!'

After documentation comes actually making the product. We have already discussed the importance of instructions and SOPs, and how and where you make the product; the next issue is who makes it. In most units, there are qualified pharmacy technicians who make the products but, as you are in this training rotation, you have to learn how to do this. This requires you to demonstrate your manual dexterity, or in my case lack of it. You have to demonstrate that you can draw up a certain volume of fluid into a syringe with no bubbles and close off the syringe with a screw cap. This may sound easy and is probably something that you did at university during chemistry or pharmaceutics practicals, but you have to add in the problem of doing the same activity in an isolator with your hands in a pair of thick gloves. Once you have got over this think about from where you are taking your liquid: is it a vial or an ampoule? If it is a vial you need to consider air pressures and how to use a venting needle; if it is an ampoule, think about snapping its neck. If you are not very good with your hands, it is worth having a set of tissues and spare gloves available when you inevitably cut your finger while trying to snap the neck of a troublesome ampoule! You have to be able to demonstrate that you can do this with consistent accuracy and with a different set of syringes and liquids.

The remaining issue for you to consider is the environment in which you make the products. If they are non-sterile products such as creams, ointments and liquids, this is fairly straightforward, but for aseptic or sterile products it can be more complicated. You need to think about cleanliness to avoid contamination. Different types of contaminant include chemical contaminants, biological contaminants and human contaminants. Chemical contaminants can arise from powders or residue left behind from previous products, biological contaminants include germs and other types of micro-organisms, and human contaminants include sweat, blood and hairs. To prevent products from becoming contaminated, you must think of all the potential risks and how they can be reduced. From your point of view this means wearing a mask and gowning up into a sterile suit properly. Again, this is not as easy as it sounds and there is an SOP explaining how it is done. Read this first, visualising what you are going to do before doing it. Pre-regs often come unstuck because they have put their gowns on and then remembered to put on the hat that covers the hair.

QUALITY ASSURANCE AND QUALITY CONTROL

Quality assurance encompasses good manufacturing practice (GMP), which can be described as aiming to ensure that products are consistently manufactured to a quality that is appropriate for their intended use. This means that the more dangerous the product to the patient, e.g. a sterile infusion for a critically ill patient, the higher the quality specification required.

None of the work that is done in any unit can be done without appropriate quality control and quality assurance support. You need to learn the difference between these and what their roles are. Some of you may have a rotation in quality control (QC), which is like going back into a lab and testing chemicals. Pre-regs can find this rotation either interesting or boring depending on what they are asked to do. The work in QC can involve testing the specifications and quality of products by drawing up specific volumes of liquid and checking their specifications such as pH and concentration. You have to use the skills that you learned from chemistry practicals at university here, so those of you who think that chemistry is irrelevant to the career of a pharmacist need to think again! You may be asked to perform environmental checks, which may include checking for biological contaminants through the use of settle plates. You may be asked to place settle plates in certain areas of the unit and then put them in the oven to allow any potential microorganisms to grow, checking to see how many and what type of organisms result.

This requires use of your microbiology knowledge, again something that you learned at university.

The role of quality assurance (QA) includes the assurance that unlicensed medicines from outside the UK are of sufficient quality for use. You may be asked to contribute to this work by chasing documentation from importing companies such as the product specification for the unlicensed medicine being imported. This can be particularly important for medicines that are licensed for different indications in their countries of origin. The product specification helps you to see if the constituent ingredients are similar to what is needed and if there are any particular ingredients that may present a problem to the patient, e.g. the amount of sugar in liquid preparations or if there is a local anaesthetic included in an injectable medicine licensed for intramuscular use which is going to be used intravenously.

Another major task that you may get involved with is with MHRA drug alerts. There are different classifications of alert, with class 1 being the most urgent. You may be asked to go to specific clinical areas to see if a particular product is on the shelves and to remove this product. To do this you need to know your way around the hospital and to have the confidence to explain to the people in charge who you are and what you are doing – after all you are taking medicines away from them. You may even be asked to go through computer records to see if such a product or batch is kept in the hospital; this may prove to be an arduous and boring task but is critically important. The worst-case scenario may be that you have to go through paper records for this information.

Although technical services is not a clinical rotation, what it does is provide you with experience of working in a technical area where attention to detail in both preparing products and documentation is critical. Think about how you could transfer this knowledge and skills into other rotations. What about working in a very busy dispensary where you are asked to dispense lots of prescriptions or check the work of others? These skills could be very useful.

Lastly, the QA department takes responsibility for ensuring the quality of unlicensed medicines coming into the hospital. You have learned from your dispensary rotations how unlicensed medicines are handled from the dispensary end, but how are they procured from suppliers in the first place? Different hospitals have different systems in place for this, depending on their size and speciality, and everything is based on the requirements of the law (the Medicines Act) and the code of ethics. Again, there is lots of documentation to complete with signatures required from the consultants and, in some cases, the chief pharmacist. In some hospitals this documentation is managed and held in MI because they may not have a QA department as such. We recommend that you try to find out how the process works in your hospital: who does what and why in case you are asked to help out with processing the documentation.

'It is good that different rotations have taught me about the role of pharmacists in different settings. In this rotation I have learnt about Section 10 of the Medicines Act and good manufacturing practice.'

'The rotation was not just making extemps. It was interesting to get to know about the manufacturing licensed unit. It was good to get to grasp the legal side of it. It was good for calculations and formulas and you got to see the other side of clinical trials that you dispense.'

TOP TIPS

- Go into technical services with an open mind; it may not be a clinical rotation but you will learn a lot
- Get used to the amount of documentation; if something is not recorded then it didn't happen!
- Think about what you learned at university that you thought you would never need; you will probably need some of that here
- Take the time to learn about the law and the regulatory bodies
- Most important of all, get involved and learn as much as you can!

Community pharmacy

11

Undertaking a placement in community pharmacy is no longer a mandatory requirement of the performance standards-based programme of the Royal Pharmaceutical Society of Great Britain (RPSGB) but many, if not most, hospitals see this as a fundamental aspect of training to be a pharmacist. The length and timings of the placements vary with each hospital and most placements tend to be between 2 and 4 weeks. The rest of this section goes through some of the more important aspects of community pharmacy placements.

FINDING A SUITABLE PLACEMENT

Many of you will have some experience of working in community pharmacy through summer placements and generally will have worked for the larger multiples. When it comes to your cross-sector placements it may be tempting to go back and work either at the same store where you have prior experience or at least for the same company; this may not always be the best thing for you and you may benefit from working somewhere completely different.

You need to check with your hospital whether you have a 2-week or a 4-week placement and when this placement is to take place. Some hospitals prefer you to find your own placements whereas others have good links with local community pharmacies and already have swap arrangements in place. In the latter instance, this obviously means that you may have little choice and have to go to that pharmacy, because the community pharmacy pre-reg may be coming to your hospital. Some hospitals offer you the flexibility of either finding a placement yourself or finding one for you; you may need to make a decision on this some months before your placement is due to start because it can take some time to search for a suitable pharmacy and then get agreement from the pharmacist to take you on.

If you are going to find your own placement, there are some things that you need to think about and discuss with your tutor. It may be convenient for you to find the closest pharmacy with the least travel time, but this may not always be the best from a training point of view. One of the first things that you need to think about is whether you would prefer to work in a multiple or an independent pharmacy. Not all multiples offer cross-sector experience because it is not a compulsory requirement of the pre-reg year, so your preferred option may be a non-starter.

A large multiple may offer you the opportunity to work within a set team from whom you get support via pre-reg training resources and a team of healthcare staff. You have to think about the size and location of the pharmacy, e.g. whether it is in a residential or a shopping area, because the customers whom you see will be very different. An independent community pharmacy offers a very different experience because the pharmacy team may be smaller and the approach to work different from that of the multiple.

If you work for a large multiple chain, the benefits are that you have set objectives to achieve and your training may be more structured. You will have the opportunity to assist with corporate initiatives, such as National No Smoking Day in March, and be exposed to trained healthcare staff as well as commercial areas in which community pharmacies provide services such as photography and perfumes. Although this may not seem like pharmacy, there are opportunities to develop and refine customer services and communication skills, so all experiences can be converted into useful learning opportunities.

In our experience, some of the problems with working in large pharmacies, particularly in city centres, is that they are very busy with a mobile population so that you do not see the same person twice and cannot see the benefits of your interventions. Also, there have been occasions when the pharmacies have assumed that you have the knowledge and skills of their own pre-reg, or of a community pre-reg, and therefore have a higher expectation of you than you do yourself. They may expect you to manage the counter or work in the dispensary on the assumption that you know what to do; you may never have encountered their computer system before, let alone know where all the stock is kept.

In an independent pharmacy, you will generally have an owner pharmacist who both runs the business and provides pharmaceutical services; you will experience how to run a business and the advantages and disadvantages of doing so. A good independent pharmacist will share their experiences with you and provide you with some useful hints and tips for running a business.

You need to think about your training needs and how much actual community pharmacy experience you have. You may have worked in the summer but did not get to do much dispensing because your role was more on the counter, so you may want to choose a community pharmacy that has a heavier dispensing workload for your placement. Alternatively, you may have little experience in community pharmacy and want to go to a pharmacy with higher over-the-counter sales so that you can gain more experience there. These are things that you need to discuss with your tutor because they can guide you in making the right decision.

As a pharmacy summer student, you would generally have experienced working over the counter and could well have completed a healthcare assistant's training course, providing you with an overview of common minor ailments encountered in community pharmacy. This may be sufficient for that stage of your career but undertaking a cross-sector placement is different – you are in training to be a pharmacist and therefore need to be able to make decisions as a pharmacist. This is a very different hat to that worn by a student. All those questions that are referred to the pharmacist are, on qualification, now referred to you.

It is important that you think seriously about what you would like to gain from your community experience and put this into objectives that you can share with your pre-reg tutor and community pharmacy tutor. The RPSGB training workbook has an excellent booklet for the cross-sector experience, which will help guide you in terms of what you may experience in community pharmacy by setting some tasks and activities for you to complete. This booklet is not exhaustive and you may not be exposed to all of the things in the workbook, depending on where you work. Completing your own objectives not only provide you with the experience of identifying and prioritising your own learning needs, but also help you to achieve the performance standards relating to your own development (A5 standards). The workbook lists performance standards specifically for community pharmacy such as the provision of emergency supplies (providing prescription-only medicines without a prescription) and you should have already identified which specific performance standards you need to be signed off for after your placement.

'The placement was of definite use to my learning; it allowed me to see a lot of things that I would never come across in hospital, such as responding to symptoms.'

'My learning was self-directed – but being in a busy pharmacy I was able to see and be involved with many aspects not found in hospital; responding to symptoms, enhanced services such as supervised methadone consumption, emergency supplies and fitting of hosiery.'

PREPARING FOR THE PLACEMENT

It is very important that you prepare properly for your experience, particularly if you do not have prior experience in community pharmacy. You would have learned some responding to symptoms and counter-prescribing skills in your undergraduate degree, and your regional pharmacy teams will provide you with study days in these areas. Depending on when these study days are and when you do your placement, you may learn about these before or after your placements. There are some very good books and learning packages, such as those from the Centre for Postgraduate Pharmacy Education (CPPE), on the market, which may help you; the RPSGB has suggested reading lists for community pharmacy and, if you have no experience or confidence in community pharmacy, you may benefit from getting one of these.

Most hospital pre-regs think that their experience in community pharmacy is all about learning the *Drug Tariff* and perhaps even the *Medicines, Ethics and Practice (MEP)* guide (RPSGB). In reality, you may find that you use the BNF as well, perhaps more so than you thought. It is worth getting a copy of the most recent *Drug Tariff* before your placement and familiarising yourself with it. You need to know what each section is and where you can find specific information because inevitably there will be some questions in the registration exam from the *Drug Tariff*. Find out how your community pharmacy makes use of the *Drug Tariff* and if they don't use it try to find out why. Many pharmacy computer systems automatically endorse prescriptions and generate orders as prescriptions are dispensed. Knowledge of prescription charges and exemptions are important but you should have already encountered this in your dispensary rotations in the hospital.

You need to look through the *MEP Guide* before your placement because it provides excellent advice and information on the legalities of practice as well as standards of service provided. You may find that you encounter situations that you have not experienced before where you do not know what to do; examples are when you have an emergency supply to make and you are not sure what constitutes an emergency supply, or when you are making a sale of emergency hormonal contraception.

In terms of the pharmacy itself, find out the working hours of the pharmacy and the hours that you have to work. Hospital pre-regs generally work a 37.5-hour week but, in community pharmacy, the premises can be open for up to 100 hours, so it is important to find out your particular shift patterns. Do note that most community pharmacies do not pay for your tea breaks as hospitals do. We have encountered many instances when pre-regs have disputed the working hours and the differences have been due to tea breaks.

You need to find out early on who will be reviewing and signing your records of evidence. In some cases locum pharmacists would be happy to review and sign these, but in other cases the tutor or the manager of the branch may want to review and sign them. It is absolutely vital for you to write up your records as you go along because, if you have a locum pharmacist for a few days, there is a chance that you may never see that person again in your placement. There is no reason whatsoever why you can't take along blank templates of your records of evidence and write them up by hand during the day; remember to make copies of the prescriptions, etc. as your hospital tutor will inevitably want to review your records as well.

'I had a really good experience. I think because I was prepared beforehand and expressed the objectives I needed to achieve I gained full benefits.'

WORKING IN THE COMMUNITY

Responding to symptoms

Pre-regs often tell us that there is more patient contact in a hospital pharmacy than in a community pharmacy. This is not the case given that about six million customers visit pharmacies every day. The difference in interpretation may be due to the differences between a patient and a customer. It is important to recognise that not everyone in community pharmacy is a patient.

To provide a broad definition, a patient is someone who has, or may have, a pre-existing medical condition whereas a customer is someone who comes to the business to purchase a service or a product; there may not be anything wrong with that person. Customers may also be called clients or consumers depending on where you work; the differences are interpretations of the same word.

Customers come to the pharmacy to buy products that may not be pharmaceutical; you will find that most pharmacy businesses rely on their non-pharmaceutical trade and you will be asked questions about these products just because you are a pharmacist. In our experience, customers have asked for a variety of things from hair colours, perfumes through to pet food and photography! 'You are a pharmacist and you sell these products so you should know all there is to know about them' is the common statement.

For a hospital pre-reg going into the community for the first time, we would recommend that you spend your first few days getting to know where everything is on the shop floor and getting to know the staff with whom you are going to work. Find out how much involvement the pharmacist has with regard to over-the-counter sales. Do they work under standard operating procedures and require you to work within these as well, and when do you refer to the pharmacist? Note that you may well be that pharmacist in a few months' time. You need to learn how the till operates and whether or not you are allowed to use it; find out if the pharmacy has a chip-and-pin machine and how to use it.

Once you have settled in, the real work starts. Our advice would be to find out which are the common minor ailments encountered in that pharmacy and start to learn about the product ranges on offer. You may want to start by learning the various product names and then looking at the constituent ingredients of these products. You need your knowledge of pharmacology here while you think about the mechanisms of action for each of the ingredients; you will find that some of the cough remedies in particular have ingredients that do not make sense, i.e. an expectorant mixed with a suppressant! Pay particular interest to the painkillers because there are a lot of them out there, each with slightly different ingredients. When you recommend a sale, try to pick the most appropriate painkiller for the patient using your knowledge of the ingredients. Some customers will not know that they must not have NSAIDs (non-steroidal anti-inflammatory drugs) if they are asthmatic and may not be aware that certain products contain NSAIDs. Check with the pharmacist why they chose a particular product; some pharmacists can answer this, others can't. Many pharmacists limit themselves to a specified range of products that they prefer to recommend because they have experience with them, but there is no real reason for not using an alternative. In this way, you can build up your knowledge and come up with your own personal product range from which you make your own recommendations.

You may get involved with minor ailment schemes and medicine use reviews (MURs), where you can apply the knowledge that you have gained and have one-to-one consultations with patients. Some pharmacists have different approaches to these; it is not unheard of for pharmacies to no longer undertake MURs because they have met their targets for the year and further MURs do not bring them any additional income. Similarly, for smoking cessation, some pharmacies do not do this because they spend a disproportionate amount of time with the patient and only get the full fee if the patient quits within a given time. Find out what your pharmacy does and what local agreements are in place with its primary care trust.

You need to identify how your pharmacist works in terms of making referrals to him or her. Some pharmacists prefer everything to be referred so that they can deal with them themselves, and you can observe and learn from them. There are others who prefer you to deal with these as part of your learning, as long as you are comfortable to do this, and keep you under supervision from a distance. There are still more pharmacists who prefer to stay behind the counter in the dispensary and provide answers to the counter staff without actually seeing the patient. You need to be flexible and learn quickly which type of pharmacist you are working with.

'Sometimes the OTC counter was not useful, so I spoke up and said that my time would be better spent checking and dispensing and if there was a patient looking to speak to a pharmacist I could take the enquiry.'

Dispensing

The interesting thing about working in the community from a hospital pharmacist's perspective is that many prescriptions are prescribed by brand name in the community. Community pharmacists are not allowed to supply anything other than what is stated on the prescription; this is a requirement of the Medicines Act. In hospital practice, it is custom and practice to contact the doctor and amend the prescription, often changing the drug itself, whereas in community pharmacy you need the doctor to provide an amended prescription. It is worth seeing the nature of the communication between pharmacist and doctor and how each professional sees the other.

Many hospital pre-regs find that they need to learn the requirements for endorsing prescriptions. In reality the process is exactly the same as in hospital because you indicate how many dose units were supplied and from what pack size. It is very important for you to read the *Drug Tariff* and familiarise yourselves with the endorsement categories. Most community pharmacies use their pharmacy computer systems to automatically endorse the prescriptions, but it remains important for you to learn what to do, not least because this is part of the syllabus for the registration exam.

It is common practice in community pharmacy not to open a sealed box and to place the dispensing label on the box; this is not done in hospital pharmacy. The labels on the medicines have to correspond exactly with the instructions on the prescription and many prescriptions are still generated with either no or incorrect instructions and the labels say 'Take as directed by the prescriber'. You should find out why this is the case from a legal point of view and how this compares with hospital practice.

One of the interesting aspects of community pharmacy is how they manage their controlled drug prescriptions. Although all pharmacies adhere strictly to the law, the way in which they do this can sometimes differ. Some pharmacies will dispense a controlled drug prescription, e.g. methadone, and enter this into the controlled drugs register when they have dispensed this, whereas others will wait for the prescription to be collected or taken by the patient before making the entry in the register. Some pharmacies even supervise the administration of methadone, which is unlikely to happen in a hospital pharmacy.

As all aspects of working in community pharmacy are covered within standard operating procedures, you need to ensure that you familiarise yourselves with them. It may be that the way you work following standard operating procedures is different to how you have been trained in hospital, although the differences may only be in the order in which you do things. You need to learn the layout of the dispensary and where everything is kept. Every pharmacy is different and, particularly for small independents, they are set up by the owner/manager so there may be some anomalies where certain things are kept. Some pharmacies keep their fast-moving lines on a separate shelf. It is useful for you to ask the pharmacist, or a locum pharmacist, how he or she copes with working in different pharmacies and if there is a system for finding out the layout of the dispensary (e.g. particular products that he or she looks out for).

You need to learn the work streams in terms of how prescriptions are processed in your pharmacy. Many pharmacies have accredited checking technicians (ACTs) who are allowed to do a final check of prescriptions once they have been clinically screened by a pharmacist. This clinical screen may be at the start or the end of the prescription. It is worth seeing the types of questions that are asked when a patient presents a prescription to the counter and comparing this with what is asked in a hospital pharmacy.

In some pharmacies you may be fortunate enough to experience difficult ethical decision-making such as emergency supplies and the supply of emergency hormonal contraception. You need to ensure that you take these opportunities to learn the law and the guidance in the code of ethics from the *MEP Guide*. Refusing an emergency supply is always difficult and it is worth discussing these issues with your pharmacists; they may all have different opinions. When you are a pharmacist, you will have your own position as to what you will accept and what you will refuse.

'My placement has made me much more aware of how community pharmacies run – would not have felt at all comfortable doing a locum in community post-registration without this placement. The RPSGB workbook was good and was easy to follow.'

'It was really useful to see the technical and logistical details of running a pharmacy which we don't see much of in the hospital.'

TOP TIPS

- Find a suitable placement for yourself
- Prepare for the placement by identifying what you specifically need to do
- Familiarise yourself with the *Drug Tariff* and the *MEP Guide*
- Be prepared to think on your feet
- Write up records of evidence as you go along and get them reviewed and signed
- Apply your learning on responding to symptoms, dispensing and the law

REFERENCES

NHS England and Wales. *Drug Tariff*. London: The Stationery Office, published monthly.

RPSGB. *Medicines, Ethics and Practice: A guide for pharmacists and pharmacy technicians*. London: Royal Pharmaceutical Society of Great Britain, published annually.

Pharmacy in the wider healthcare environment

12

Your pre-reg programme may have some scope to show you areas of pharmacy- and non-pharmacy-related areas to put your own practice into perspective with other pharmacy staff who have specialist expertise, or with other healthcare professionals. It is useful to have a different viewpoint about what we do as pharmacists in order to avoid becoming blinkered. Pharmacy has its place within the wider healthcare picture and is certainly not the be all and end all. It is also useful to realise that hospital pharmacy is not the only route that your career can take and, even if it is the route that you will be taking in the near future, knowing whom and where to contact inside and outside the hospital will help you in your job.

You may have the opportunity to spend some time with more experienced or specialist members of your pharmacy team. These are useful insights into the possible pathways that you could follow in your future career. Be sure to ask about the career path of your specialist practitioners, because you may be surprised at the winding road that they took to get where they are now. Be careful to keeps things in perspective though, because a lot of hard work is needed to become a specialist practitioner – it certainly does not happen overnight.

In addition, do not get too carried away about visiting and shadowing every conceivable person or clinic. Remember that, for your pre-reg year, the best way of learning is by 'doing'. You will have a job getting to grips with basic pharmacy practice and the more common medical conditions, without even touching on the more complicated issues.

When attending non-pharmacy-related activities, you need to question the relevancy of what you are doing. Saying this, shadowing a nurse on the medication round or sitting in on a prescribing clinic can give you useful insight into the thought processes of different healthcare professionals and the problems that they face. It is useful to get perspectives on medicines from other healthcare professionals because you may be surprised how much they know about medicines – or how little, even if they are working with medicines on a daily basis.

PRIMARY CARE TRUSTS

It is useful if you get the opportunity to visit your local primary care trust (PCT) because this gives you a wider perspective on how your local health-care system works. Different PCTs work differently and are staffed with a range of pharmacy and non-pharmacy staff.

Please see the section on specialist PCT placement in Section 6 for more general information on PCTs. The quotes here identify many of the experiences that pre-regs have had and the range of tasks with which they have been involved.

'I was able to grasp an understanding of the different roles of pharmacists within the PCT through working with various members of the team on different tasks. This included analysing ePACT data and feeding back to GP practices for areas of change, reviewing recently produced NICE guidelines and highlighting any issues relevant to primary care, education and training of healthcare professionals in the PCT, including community pharmacists, nurses and GPs. Through visiting the GP practice I was able to see the roles of various healthcare professionals working in the practice.'

'Analysing ePACT data and attending the prescription review and discussion with the prescribing review pharmacist enabled me to learn about the prescribing issues in the local area; some of these included prescribing brand name drugs when a therapeutically equivalent generic product was available, over-prescribing of antibiotics and reviewing patients on medicines that are to be withdrawn next year.'

'I now have a better overall understanding of how healthcare is delivered in the community and the role of various healthcare professionals in delivering these services. This will improve my communication skills when dealing with professionals in the community while I am working in hospital. Also I will be able to advise patients in hospital as to the services available to them out in the community and also advise other professionals in the hospital where they can signpost patients to. I now have a greater ability to analyse documents and highlight the key points; this may improve my skills when working in areas of hospital pharmacy such as medicines information. Also my presentation skills have improved as I delivered a presentation to a group

of colleagues and answered their questions. If I return to PCT or community
pharmacy I already have basic skills needed to perform in that job.'

'During my PCT placement, I attended team meetings, went on various
visits, spent time reading and interpreting DH documents and gained a
comprehensive understanding of the role of a pharmacist within the PCT.
I have learnt that PCT pharmacists have a crucial role in commissioning
services and controlling budget to ensure that the health needs of their
particular community is met. They also act as a valuable source of advice
with regard to prescribing guidelines, treatment strategies and impact on
primary care.'

'By attending visits I learnt the importance of building a rapport with patients
from all walks of life and strategies to do this. I also gained an appreciation of
the pharmacist's role within these different care settings as well as allied
healthcare professionals, and how in the end the healthcare team needs to
work together efficiently, to ensure the best outcome for the patients.'

'I saw, first hand, how complicated some NICE guidelines are especially for
busy healthcare professionals who need information at their finger tips that is
accessible and user friendly I therefore bore this in mind while producing
summary sheets.'

'Through attending the PCT team meeting and reading various DH papers
such as the new contractual framework for community pharmacy, *A Vision
for Pharmacy*, *Standards for Better Health*, *Medicines Matters* and *Our
Health, Our Care, Our* Say, I learned about the changes in pharmacy at
the moment and how PCTs have a key role in this. They were focused on
the importance of bringing and delivering care to the community, ensuring
better access to services and promoting health not just treating the sick. I also
realised that key to all of this is the integration and cooperation of community
pharmacists with other healthcare professionals, and ensuring that a wider
range of services is available in the community itself.'

'I have gained an important understanding of the role of the PCT in budgeting
and prescribing decisions made; with this in mind I found it useful to see the
process of how a medication is prescribed from the very top end. More
specifically I can see why prescribing decisions have been made rather than
simply reacting to them; this will in turn help me when I receive a prescription
to understand the thought process behind why a medication has been prescribed. I have also seen how important it is to provide services specific to the
community and specific to patients themselves rather than generically; this
will help my practice as a whole. On my visits I learnt how to communicate
better with patients and gain their trust; this will be invaluable and I look
forward to applying these skills in my practice. I also learnt the importance of
a smooth and efficient interaction between primary and secondary care and

how all healthcare professionals including pharmacists have a responsibility to ensure that it is well maintained.'

'This placement has emphasised to me the role of a pharmacist as an expert in medicines, and how this knowledge can be used when working as an integrated team in primary care. My knowledge of services available in the community has improved and this will enable me to provide advice and signpost patients that I encounter in hospital more appropriately. I have enhanced my appreciation of clarity of information given to others and also in assessing patients individually when help is needed with compliance with medication. This placement has been extremely valuable and worthwhile. I have developed my understanding of the healthcare structure and especially the role of PCTs.'

PRISON PHARMACY

Prison pharmacy is a specialist area worth visiting. You may have some preconceived ideas about what prison life, and prisoners, are like. But, at the end of the day, they are people who need access to healthcare just like anyone else. Find out where your local prison is and what type of healthcare they provide for the prisoners. Remember that there are security issues with entering a prison that must be adhered to.

Visiting a prison will give you insight in terms of what your beliefs are. On visiting a prison pharmacy, many people ask questions about whether prisoners 'deserve' the healthcare to which they have access. It is useful to think about all the ethical and professional issues that come with working in a prison, and this may help you to define the limits of your practice.

Rather than describe some of what you may expect from visiting a prison pharmacy, we thought some comments from our pre-regs would be just as good.

'I discussed with pharmacists and technicians their role within the prison. A large majority of what they do is similar to in a community pharmacy. A pharmacist's role is to provide advice to the patients in a minor ailment clinic conducted in the morning and prescribe any necessary interventions, and check dispensed items. The lead pharmacist in the prison also takes on a managerial role for the pharmacy and reviews procedures in place for the delivery of pharmacy services within the prison environment and implements any necessary changes. The technician's role includes dispensing accurately the medications on the prescription and performing stock checks.'

'Other healthcare professionals working in the prison include GPs, physiotherapists, dentists and radiographers. They come into the prison and care for the patients who need their services as they would outside the prison. Nurses in the prison are responsible for delivering medicines to patients and conducting clinics. Specialist nurses from a substance misuse team see patients with drug addictions and review the control of their addiction within the prison environment, with the ultimate aim of withdrawing patients from their illegal drug use entirely.'

'The main prescribing issues were around substance misuse. It was often difficult to assess the amount of methadone or Subutex a patient should be on, as they might lie about their use outside or inside the prison. Other drugs such as benzodiazepines also have the potential for abuse either by the patient themselves or they may trade to other prisoners. I now have a greater understanding of substance misuse, which I can apply should I come across a substance misuse patient again.'

'Medicines, which are kept on the wing, are safely secured in a locked cupboard. It was debatable whether or not the patient should be in possession of their own medication; they were assessed to see if it was safe for them to have their medication in their own possession. Some patients would be made to take their medicines under supervision. Patients may be given a supply of their medication for their own possession on a daily, weekly or monthly basis based on the safety assessment.'

'From reading *A Pharmacy Service for Prisons* I learnt about the problems in providing healthcare in prison and the vision for how healthcare should be delivered in prisons. The ultimate aim is to provide prisoners with the same access to healthcare they would have in the community. Changes have been made in the prison in order to improve pharmacy services.'

'It was very interesting to see pharmacy in a completely different environment and look at the issues in delivering pharmacy services in such an environment. It has given me a broader look on the types of patients with their various issues that you may come across in pharmacy. It was also good to get an insight into the realities of prison life.'

'I have learnt that even though there is a stigma surrounding prison healthcare and treating the prisoners – they actually are *people* that require our professional help and expertise. I won't let personal beliefs or other people's beliefs cloud my judgement (professionally speaking) in providing healthcare to any person seeking it. I feel that this is a core tenet of professionalism – and something I will carry for the rest of my life. This was an amazing experience overall. At first I didn't know what to expect but then warmed into it well.

I enjoyed speaking to and shadowing other healthcare staff. I also enjoyed interacting with the prisoners – by speaking to them it puts colour into the full healthcare picture. All pharmacy staff were incredibly friendly and I would most definitely consider this type of work in my future career.'

'This enjoyable experience showed me the integrated network of healthcare provided for the prisoners, e.g. outreach, mental health, substance misuse, GPs. I was amazed at the types of services provided by the pharmacy team such as minor ailments and smoking cessation. The pharmacist was also involved in setting up medication systems to allow prisoners to keep possession of their meds. I learned how meds are distributed and about funding for prison healthcare. The experience helped me to realise the importance of being non-judgemental towards the public. I learned that building a rapport with the prisoners gained their respect. I also learned that pharmacists can help to improve general health of the prisoners by providing additional services. In the future, I will always aim to use my initiative to set up services such as self-help groups or chronic disease management.'

'Probably one of the best experiences of my pre-reg year so far. It was great to see the pharmacy team playing such an important role in the healthcare system, particularly in the area of substance misuse. Prison pharmacy is definitely an area I would consider getting involved in when I qualify and this placement has given me the chance to discover this.'

TOP TIPS

- If you can, get as much experience of members of the wider healthcare team
- Find out what they understand to be the role of the pharmacist
- Find out about the roles of PCT pharmacists and how they influence both primary and secondary care prescribing
- Find out what other areas in healthcare primary care pharmacists get involved with
- Have an open mind when visiting a prison pharmacy; the prisoners are people who need access to healthcare
- Compare and contrast how services are provided in a prison with what you have already experienced

Section 3

Assessment and feedback

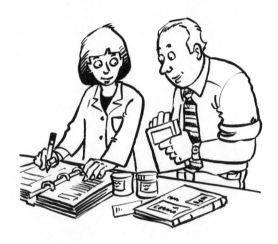

Assessment and feedback: how to get through these

13

'When does all of this assessment ever stop?'
'When am I going to know that I can finally do something properly?'
'How do I know that I am doing something right?'
'I need some feedback about how to improve and all I keep getting is how well I am doing.'

The comments in the box are just some of the ones that we always receive from pre-regs during the year. You are assessed on all aspects of your work during the year, both formally and informally. A wide range of people assess you including your supervising pharmacists, pharmacists with whom you work as well as pharmacy technicians in both the ward and the dispensary; anybody and everybody can be involved with your assessments. Assessment is one of the most important aspects of the pre-reg year with which you have to get to grips because it shouldn't actually matter who undertakes your assessment as long as they are capable of assessing you. In our experience, not everyone can undertake assessments, which often presents some problems for you.

Although most of the assessments use the Royal Pharmaceutical Society of Great Britain (RPSGB) performance standards, sometimes you are assessed against internal standards set by the supervising pharmacists or pharmacy technicians. The problem is that initially you may not know what these are. Your task is to start each rotation with a view to working with different people who prefer to work in different ways. This can range from when you are working on the wards and your pharmacist likes you to record medication histories in a certain way, to speaking to the patient about medicines using a certain sequence of questions. If you deviate from this you will be spoken to! Alternatively, it is not uncommon to find out that you must dispense a certain type of medicine (e.g. a liquid) on a certain bench. Labelling of medicines can present enormous difficulties; just exactly where do you stick the label on the box?

The whole aspect of assessment during the pre-reg year can vary depending on at which hospital you work, how many staff they have and who is responsible for training. It is important not to compare what happens at one hospital with what happens at another, although, if you have had no sort of assessment well into your pre-reg year, you should take action by speaking in the first instance to your tutor. Some hospitals have their own dedicated paperwork for each type of assessment whereas others have no paperwork at all. Remember that you need to provide some sort of evidence for your tutor so, even if an assessment is an informal one, it is well worth having a written record of this. You may have to write a record of evidence about your assessment if your assessor does not have the time to complete one at the time.

In some hospitals you may find that your supervisor is new to pre-reg training and does not know exactly what to do and how to complete any paperwork. You may need to guide that person through this, so you need to familiarise yourself with the assessment paperwork first. You may also find that your supervisor does not really know your level of knowledge and starts to ask questions that are either too easy or too difficult. If they are too easy this is an opportunity for you to demonstrate your knowledge, but if too difficult you can learn from this by thinking about why you are being asked what you are being asked, and where you can find the answers.

ASSESSMENT IN THE DISPENSARY

In the dispensary, the main types of assessment involve the activities in the list below and all hospitals have similar types. The activities are all assessed and feedback given during your dispensary rotations; the assessment often involves doing dispensary tests of a certain format, usually using a range of prescriptions, and having to complete in a limited timeframe. The feedback for this assessment is given to you by your dispensary trainer in a formal manner. Each of the aspects assesses both your knowledge and your skills in:

- Labelling
- Dispensing
- Screening
- Checking
- Patient counselling.

When generating labels, different pharmacists have their own preferences for instructions on the labels and how they are written; this is particularly so when the instructions are free format and those labelling can write what they want. The trick is to learn what each pharmacist prefers and be flexible in line with this. The whole issue of where exactly to stick the label on the box is a very serious one; you will be in hot water if the label is in the wrong place!

In terms of dispensing and checking, this is all about sticking the right label on the right box with the right instructions; this sounds very easy but in reality many pre-regs can't do this at the start of their year. You will find yourself making many excuses when it's your turn to make these mistakes, so be careful to check that the excuses have stood the test of time. Think about what you learned at university during pharmacy practice classes and the dispensing tests that you had to pass. At university you may have had an hour or so to complete one prescription; in the workplace this may be limited to a few minutes to complete a similar prescription.

The common errors that pre-regs make are no different to those that are widely known about and documented. From our own dispensing assessments we found that the range of errors NOT picked up included the following:

- Out-of-date product
- Labels of two containers swapped over
- Missing patient information leaflet
- Incorrect length of treatment
- Incorrect quantity
- Wrong strength
- Incorrect instructions
- When required versus regular labels
- Incorrect route of administration
- Incorrect product supplied.

The advice that we gave to the pre-regs at the time was to remind them of the points in the box.

'Remember, if you have not scored 100%, you will have to re-sit, since **any checking error breaches the Medicines Act** and means that you have therefore committed an illegal act.'

'Some consideration will be given to those pre-regs who have not completed their checking log.'

'In any case, if you have not passed this test, you will need to re-sit it, so that your tutor can then be able to sign you off performance standard "**C1.12 Effectively check prescriptions checked by others**".'

'If you have already been signed off, then **your tutors will "un-sign"** this **performance standard** until you can competently demonstrate that you can check without errors. Considering that, in 3 months' time you will all be registered pharmacists, checking prescriptions without errors should be the LEAST that you can do.'

Screening, or clinical screening, can be called different things in different hospitals but is essentially the same process. It includes undertaking a technical check to ensure that all the legal aspects of a prescription are present, then a clinical check to see if the drugs, doses and frequencies are consistent with the patient's condition. The major issues with clinical screening include making assumptions about the prescriptions or the patients that may be incorrect or inappropriate, e.g. assuming that the patient has had a particular medication before or would know how to use a particular drug or device. Screening is hard at the best of times, because you may not always understand the patient's clinical diagnosis or the surgical procedure that has to be done before you can put the medicines into context. You may now know enough about some of the medicines themselves to identify whether or not they are appropriate. This is something that you will find during your dispensary assessments because some of the prescriptions are set up for you to think about these issues.

One of the more common informal ways of feedback is when someone says loudly to no one in particular 'Who was it who dispensed this prescription?'. Someone else says that it was 'the pre-reg', with the response 'Where is that pre-reg?'; it goes on from there. This form of feedback, although not always appropriate, is so common that you will definitely experience it at some point during your dispensary rotation. You may be lucky enough not to be that pre-reg; the conversation may not relate to pre-regs and can equally be applied to junior pharmacists or pharmacy technicians. In some cases the pre-reg is always the first one to be blamed, especially if you have a 'hit or miss' approach to your dispensing.

ASSESSMENT ON THE WARDS

Assessments on the wards are very different to the dispensary experience, and every clinical pharmacist will want to assess you first before they let you loose to speak to patients, doctors and nurses. The assessments can cover a range of activities and, depending on where you work, you may be assessed in each activity separately before you move on to the next stage. Your hospital will have a number of assessment tools and checklists already in place for pharmacists, and you may be assessed using the same tools and checklists. These cover activities such as medication history taking, patient consultations and general working on the wards.

Reading through a set of medical notes and relating these to the current prescription is one of the first activities to be assessed. Although many of you have done this at university, you quickly find that in real life a set of clinical notes is generally all over the place with nothing where it should be. At university your clinical notes would have been clear and sequential with entries all appearing in date order; you may even be able to read the doctor's handwriting!

Screening medication charts or discharge prescriptions forms a big part of ward-based pharmacy and the process is much the same as that used for clinical screening in the dispensary. The main difference is that you have other resources on the ward that you don't have in the dispensary, namely the patient, the notes and the healthcare staff. You also have the patients' medications if they brought them in, so can compare what patients came in on with what they are taking and what they will go home with. Assessments that you may experience on the wards involve accompanying your supervising pharmacists on ward visits, when you are expected to go through the patients' medication charts and their medications, justifying why each is being used. You have to have a thorough knowledge of why these medicines are there, how they work and what you need to monitor.

One of the problems is that you may know how medicines work theoretically from your studies at university, but this may be at a molecular or receptor level, whereas what is needed on the ward is a practical and pragmatic knowledge of how medicines work. This is not to say that the molecular level is not important, just that you have to communicate how the medicines work to the patient who may not understand the technical words that you use.

When monitoring medicines, this includes the side effects in addition to other monitoring requirements such as blood results and therapeutic levels. It is usual for pre-regs to say that the side effects of most drugs are nausea, vomiting and diarrhoea; indeed this is often the default position for many pre-regs when asked this question. It is also common for pre-regs to state that they will monitor the urea and electrolytes without specifying which ones and what they would expect to see.

Speaking with patients is one of the more stressful things that you will encounter, simply because a pharmacist, or a pharmacy technician, observes you as you talk to the patient. You have had training on how to take a medication history and what questions to ask to establish what medicines a patient takes, but in real life things do not always work like that!

'I get nervous when I start talking to patients, especially when someone is watching me. In my first drug history I was very nervous and had the checklist with me so that I could go through it. I asked the patient all of the questions I thought were needed and concentrated on the questions relating to complementary medicines, smoking and alcohol as I always forget these and wrote all of these down neatly in my notebook to show to the pharmacist. When she read what I had written, she asked me where the patient's current medicines were. I was gob smacked, in my nervousness I had forgotten to ask the patient about his current medicines and had only focused on the questions that I was not confident with. I had to go back and ask the patient what medicines he currently took. I was really embarrassed.'

Speaking to doctors can be frightening at first, but it becomes easier as you realise that they are sometimes asking because they don't know themselves. When it comes to assessing how you speak to doctors, much inevitably depends on how your supervising pharmacist thinks you should talk to them. Some pharmacists prefer to have a relatively informal relationship with junior doctors and a more formal relationship with consultants; others prefer to keep everything formal. You need to find out what your supervising pharmacist's preferred style is. Most of the assessment for this is informal and based on your everyday practice. If the pharmacist feels that you become nervous before speaking to doctors, you might need to work on this. It may just be that you are nervous because you are worried that they will ask you a question to which you don't know the answer. You need to learn the skill of being able to say that you don't know something with confidence; doctors don't worry that they don't know something because they can always ask.

Speaking to other staff on the ward is not generally a problem and most of you will be fine speaking to nurses and other healthcare staff. Again, this is not something that is assessed formally but it is worth noting that nurses often know a lot about the patient and the medicines that they are taking. They may not always know why certain medicines are being used or how to administer parenteral medicines, but they know a great deal. You may be assessed on how you explain to a nurse what a medicine is being used for or how to administer a particular parenteral medicine. Ward-based teaching is very common and may be one of the things on which you are assessed.

ASSESSMENT IN MI

The most common assessments in medicines information (MI) relate to how you answer the phone and how you construct your enquiries. In terms of answering the phone, it is all about how you ask questions of the enquirer and how well you listen in order to capture the relevant pieces of information being provided. It is often the case that either the enquirer provides too little information for you to have a proper context for the enquiry or there is so much information that you don't know what is and is not important. Your supervising pharmacist will listen to how you answer the phone and what you ask, as well as how you ask, during the early stages of your rotation, although he or she may keep his or her head down so as not to put you off. Once you have been formally 'signed off' on answering the phone, your supervising pharmacist will let you answer when the phone rings and leave you to it.

The ability to construct an answer to an enquiry can be a little more tricky, and you should have read through and applied what you have learned from the UKMI workbook. Your supervising pharmacist goes through your workbook and your answers before allowing you to answer enquiries on your own. This is one of the assessments to ensure that you are not using the wrong reference sources or going off on a tangent. The process of answering an enquiry is very systematic and robust, and you are assessed on how well you followed that process. It is important to embed the process into your work practice.

Most of the feedback that you receive from MI is instantaneous because you are working alongside your supervising pharmacist and going through your enquiries together before giving the response. The feedback provides you with some direction and advice on what other reference sources may be useful, which is the supervisor's way of assessing how well you follow the processes of answering an enquiry. The speed at which you progress through your rotation may be another indication of how well you are doing, because a supervisor will not allow you to answer the phone unless you can do it and also won't give you complex enquiries to answer.

ASSESSMENT IN TECHNICAL SERVICES

Technical services is a very controlled rotation and you are formally assessed in everything that you do. You will find that there is a standard operating procedure for everything, even how to wash your hands, and you need to read this and sign that you have read it. The range of activities on which you are assessed includes:

- Hand washing
- Preparing trays for making products
- Preparing worksheets from prescriptions
- Recording batch numbers and expiry dates in worksheets
- Gowning up
- Recording of environmental monitoring
- Undertaking broth runs to assess aseptic technique

- The law in relation to Section 10 of the Medicines Act
- Calculations.

Many of the above assessments are obvious and fairly straightforward although there are a few that traditionally cause pre-regs some problems. In our experience the main ones are gowning up and undertaking broth runs. These can be demonstrated by the comments in the box.

'I thought I knew how to gown up as I had read the SOP thoroughly and was going through it step by step. When I thought I was ready I realised that I had forgotten to put on the hat underneath the hood and now it was too late and I had to start again!'

'The broth run was going really well until I realised that I was not wearing the right sized gloves because they were too small and tight. I thought that I would carry on but while I was thinking about what to do with the gloves I had a little accident and spilt some of the broth on the bench. I quickly cleaned it up and then I was worried that I would fail the test because I did not have enough broth to fill all of the bottles.'

'I'm not very good with my hands and am always spilling things and cutting myself; I was really worried that I would do this during the test but I concentrated really hard and took much longer than I had expected. Time ran away from me and I didn't realise that I had been in the unit for all of the morning and everyone had gone to lunch when I came out.'

TOP TIPS

- Assessment is really important; be honest with yourself and your supervisors
- Try to accept negative/constructive criticism and use this as positive criticism to strengthen your weaknesses
- It is unlikely that you will be good at everything in the pre-reg year; everyone has their weaknesses

Getting signed off: how do you know you are there?

As you are probably aware by now, during your year you are assessed and receive feedback most of the time in a variety of ways. The question then is how to convince your tutor that you can be signed off for the performance standards. Before we discuss some of the formal reviews it is a good time to discuss what we mean by 'being signed off'.

Your tutor has to sign each performance standard where you have consistently met the minimum competence required for that standard; the minimum requirement tends to vary depending on the tutor, the hospital and even the performance standard itself. What we mean here is that you may need to prove yourself against performance standards many times during the year (e.g. managing your time effectively), whereas for other standards such as 'managing conflict' you may be able to provide evidence for this just once or twice.

Why do we say that the minimum requirement depends on the tutor and hospital? Well, each tutor has his or her own expectations of what is required and it is up to you to find out what is needed. In terms of the hospital, this depends on how your training programme is structured and whether there are further opportunities to demonstrate your competence in other rotations. An example of this may be that you have completed your patient services training in the dispensary but are still not that confident at checking other people's dispensing; your tutor may therefore ask you to provide more evidence from your community pharmacy placement. If, on the other hand, you have completed all of the rotations where you will be dispensing your tutor may decide to sign you off. In most cases, signing you off is a joint decision between you and your tutor, and you have the option to say that you do not want to be signed off; strange as it may sound, we have certainly had pre-regs who asked not to be signed off because they did not feel quite ready.

We now go through some of the more formal reviews such as end-of-rotation reviews and the more formal Royal Pharmaceutical Society of Great Britain (RPSGB) progress reviews.

END-OF-ROTATION REVIEWS

At the end of each rotation, and often in the middle of rotations too, you should expect to have some kind of assessment by your rotation supervisor. Do not expect this always to be a pharmacist, because in some highly technical areas it may be entirely appropriate for technical staff to appraise you.

Each hospital has a different system but there should be some paperwork involved in your rotation appraisals – which is in whatever format your rotation or hospital chooses to use. If you need to fill in paperwork before your meeting, please ensure that you do so, so that you can make the most of this review meeting.

Please remember that it should be YOUR responsibility to ensure that you have a review in each rotation. Although your primary aim is to gain skills and experience in that rotation, bear in mind that your supervisor will have a million other things to do and seeing you may not be uppermost in his or her thoughts. Your supervisor may be responsible for delivery of pharmacy services, and there may be other student or trainee groups in the same area as you who need his or her time. Therefore it is up to YOU to set up an end-of-rotation review meeting and for YOU to provide your supervisor with all the evidence that you have gathered while in the rotation, so that he or she can then quickly and easily make a judgement on which performance standards you have demonstrated competency in.

Expect your supervisor to deem you to be competent in his or her areas. This does not mean that your tutor will then sign you off as being competent, however, because your tutor will have a wider perspective on your performance over the whole training year and may think that you can demonstrate those same performance standards in a different rotation. So, don't get too excited when your rotation supervisor signs you off as being competent in lots of performance standards, because your tutor may not see things the same way.

RPSGB PROGRESS REVIEWS

Although you may visit your tutor on a regular basis, every 13 weeks you meet more formally with your tutor to undertake the RPSGB 13-week progress review. These meetings are very important, because, in these meetings, you and your tutor decide which performance standards you are competent in, and submit this on formal paperwork to the RPSGB for their records. At these progress reviews, you and your tutor have to make a judgement about how well you are progressing, and make plans on how to successfully cover the remaining performance standards.

Review at 13 weeks

Thirteen weeks will fly by very quickly and you will be at the 13-week progress review before you know it. You may feel at this time that you have not demonstrated competency in many areas. This is because you have probably been spending time just familiarising yourself with your surroundings and the different ways of working in your hospital, and generally getting used to coming to work! At this time, you should not realistically expect to be signed off many performance standards, even if you have quite a lot of evidence from your rotations so far. You may be confused as to what standard your tutor is judging your performance by – the best way to think about it is: 'Can I perform this performance standard to the standard that would be expected of a newly qualified pharmacist?' If the answer is no, you should not expect your tutor to sign you off! Another issue might be whether your tutor thinks that you can demonstrate particular performance standards better in your other rotations. Although you may have ably demonstrated that you can dispense at ward level, for example, it might be better to reserve judgement on your dispensing skills until you complete your rotation in dispensary.

Review at 26 weeks

By 26 weeks you should expect to have gathered a fair amount of evidence. You also should have rotated through enough rotations to get a feel for what is happening in your hospital pharmacy department, and have more of a grasp of what is expected from you in terms of evidence to demonstrate your competence.

Although you are halfway through your year, you may not be 'halfway there' in terms of performance standards. In our many years of experience as tutors, we would expect that most pre-regs perform best (in terms of fulfilling a greater number of performance standards) between 13 and 39 weeks, but mostly between 26 and 39 weeks.

Between 26 and 39 weeks is when you should try to hit as many performance standards as possible. This is probably where the main bulk of the evidence of your competency will be provided, as you start to make sense of the disparate rotations that you have been doing, and put together all the pieces that you have been given to construct your own practice. You should find that each rotation gets easier and easier in terms of settling in, and you might make more of the rotations that are in the middle and towards the end of the year, and everything starts to make much more sense!

During this time, try to think seriously about how well you are getting on with your calculations because, by 39 weeks, you should be consistently getting 80% on calculation tests or you risk not being entered for the registration exam.

Review at 39 weeks

Your 39-week progress review is a very important meeting with your tutor, because this is where you and your tutor decide whether you can fulfil the remaining performance standards by the end of your training. If your performance is NOT satisfactory this should have been flagged up before the 39-week progress review so that it doesn't come as a shock that arrangements may need to be made to substantially change the remainder of your training programme, to ensure more opportunities for demonstrating your competency in areas identified as being deficient or to undertake additional weeks of training.

Ideally, by 39 weeks you need to have attained most of your performance standards. This ensures that your remaining 13 weeks are as stress free as possible. For your remaining time, you then obviously need to target your activities to meet your remaining performance standards. You can also start to think about registration exam revision.

'After Easter I felt more in control of what was going on. It's all coming together. This feeling that I have that I am "on top of the game" has to become my normal minimal level of practice.'

Compared with community pharmacy, you are expected to submit a lot of written records of evidence along with logs of what you have completed, testimonials from your colleagues and rotation appraisal paperwork. This is because it is highly unlikely that your tutor was working with you for much of your pre-reg, which means that your tutor relies on this written work to make a judgement as to whether to sign you off in any performance standard. If you do turn up to these crucial meetings without the required evidence to hand, you should fully expect your tutor to refuse to sign you off.

Be careful not to make comparisons with your fellow pre-regs on how many or for which performance standards you have been signed off. Such a comparison serves no purpose, because the opportunities that you have been given to demonstrate your competence are entirely different to those of someone in a different area of pharmacy, and depend on which rotations you have done. You would reasonably expect a pre-reg in dispensary to provide evidence for different performance standards from, say, another pre-reg in MI or technical services.

In community pharmacy there is arguably a smaller range of activities for demonstrating your competence, so community tutors may sign off performance standards at an earlier stage than in a hospital. You may find that friends and colleagues doing their pre-reg in community pharmacy are having performance standards signed off quicker than you. You shouldn't worry about this because you should have all of yours signed off by the end of the year; it is not a race!

Many pre-regs enter their pre-registration training with thoughts only of the registration examination at the end of the year; unfortunately this is not the only thing that you need to worry about! The exam is just one day; the remainder of your assessment is based on evaluation of your performance throughout the year.

The difference between university and pre-registration training is that you have to remember that it is YOUR responsibility to think about your own learning needs and make the best use of the learning opportunities presented to you. This means that, in addition to learning, it is also your responsibility to demonstrate that you know how to do things, evidence of which can take the form of records of evidence.

Your pre-reg tutor, in discussion with you, is the person who makes the final assessment of competent demonstration of each performance standard as required by the RPSGB. This means that all the feedback that your tutor gets from your rotations adds to the body of evidence showing that you are competent.

By the time you have your Progress Report 3 at 39 weeks into your training, you should be fairly used to being assessed in this way. The difference with the 39-week progress review is that this is the crunch point, where some important decisions have to be made. First, you and your tutor need to look at the remaining performance standards that have still to be achieved. At this point, you both have to decide whether these are achievable in the remaining time. If so, you and your tutor can make the decision to enter you for the exam.

'I will be competent by the end of the year. When I started I felt I had no knowledge. Over the year, I know what I don't know. I know I won't kill you. A lot of clinical knowledge is still to be developed but I know about the danger signals. I know that I will prevent harm and be safe.'

If your tutor decides that your performance is NOT satisfactory, this is where there can be a problem. To be honest, you need to have had discussions with your tutor before your 39-week progress review, because it is not helpful if this kind of feedback is left until this point; you do not then have sufficient time and opportunity to do anything about the situation. If your performance has not been satisfactory, you have not been able to improve your performance and your tutor feels that you won't make the necessary improvements by the end of your training, you may be able to extend your training. In any case, you and your tutor should discuss the situation closely with the RPSGB pre-registration division, so that everyone is clear on what needs to be done.

The closer you get, the more unprepared you feel! The more you've learned, the more you realise what you don't know. Many of you will go through a rollercoaster ride of thinking whether or not you are competent, which may depend on whether you are good at, or enjoy, your current rotation! Remember that you are not expected to be brilliant at everything that you do, but to carry out things to a minimum standard as defined by the RPSGB.

When you near the stage that you have to start to take responsibility for your actions, this is when you will start to get anxious, because you then feel the weight of responsibility that a newly qualified pharmacist has to shoulder. This results in some strange circumstances. For instance, those patients on the ward that took you half an hour to deal with as a pre-reg suddenly takes you all morning and all your lunch break to sort out, and you have to pop in just before you go home just to double triple check everything! Somehow, when your signature counts for something you will make sure that absolutely everything that you sign and put your name to is absolutely correct.

Socrates said, 'The more I learn, the more I learn how little I know' and I think that this applies here. The more you've learned, the more you realise how much more there is to learn, and sometimes this can be scary – especially when patients' wellbeing and safety are at stake.

'In terms of the dispensary I'm almost there. Clinical is yet to come. I feel more confident in the dispensary. Before my hospital placement I would have rated myself 3–4 out of 10. Now I am 7 out of 10. If I work for 10 years maybe then can say I'm a 9 out of 10. I may never be "competent".'

'Yes. Competent is difficult word. One year is probably not enough time to become competent. In terms of qualifying and sitting the exam then yes I am ready.'

'Yes. I know that I can do it. I know my limitations as a pharmacist. If I don't know something, I will check and find out the answer or refer. I will always make sure I keep the patients' best interest as a priority and not to place them in danger.'

'Am I ready to be a pharmacist by July? Some days I feel ready, some days not. When I'm in a situation where I don't know what to do then I feel like I'm not ready. I would rate myself as 6.5/10 in terms of being a pharmacist. In the beginning of the year I would now rate myself as 2–3/10 but I am sure that at the time, I would have thought that I was a 5/10. The application of what you've learnt is a whole new ball game. It's the skills that matter not the knowledge.'

Final progress review

By the time that you have your final progress review it will be week 50 and you will have sat the registration exam and be in your final couple of weeks of pre-reg training. This progress review is generally quite easy because the decision to sign you off has been implicitly made between you and your tutor, and it is just a matter of completing the paperwork. A word of warning though, because if your performance has significantly dropped off in the last 13 weeks of your training the tutor reserves the right to withdraw, or un-sign, performance standards and to refuse to sign you off. This is rare but can, and does, happen.

The only other time when the 50-week review counts for something is if you have a particular rotation towards the end of your year and you have not been able to demonstrate your competence in that area. A typical example is in the dispensary where you may not have the chance to complete everything that is required and your tutor may wait until the last possible opportunity to allow you maximum time to demonstrate your competence. If this is the case you will have discussed this in your 39-week progress review.

Having said that, the final appraisal is just about completing the paperwork; we always ask our pre-regs if they are happy for us to sign them off onto the register and many of them still hesitate before saying yes! This is because they realise how much responsibility and accountability they will have as fully qualified pharmacists. We also always ask what it is that patients, and the general public, want from a pharmacist first and foremost – we leave it for you to figure out the response that we are looking for (there is a hint from one of our pre-regs below!).

'I'm ready but not ready. I've covered pretty much everything but I don't have enough experience. Previously there have always been seniors to refer to. Now it's down to me. That's what is worrying. I have to make sure that what I do is safe for patients. If I really don't know then I'll just ask. If I'm on my own in community pharmacy I'll decide myself based on judgement based on what the problem is. Should I be signed off as competent? Yes. Even if you qualify you will still forget what you've learnt and what you should do. Maybe you are never competent. I am scared now. I want to work part time in community and hospital. I don't think I have enough experience in a ward environment. My experience of community was that no one tells you that you should be confident in your behaviour and look things up. In hospital – you are told that you are more than capable as a pharmacist, you just have to believe. I had previously never treated myself as an adult. I've changed since I came here: now I'm not scared about telling people that I don't know.'

'Before I didn't have a lot of experience. Now I think about the patient, not just the process. Now I would look at the patient not just the prescription. Do I feel like a pharmacist? I feel like I *could* be a pharmacist. I feel like I use the right processes, although I can still be a bit slow. I am quite cautious. I always look things up if I'm not sure. Hopefully I am dispensing safely.'

'I am still feeling anxious. The responsibility of being a pharmacist is dawning on me now! Being a good pharmacist is not the point; being safe is more important.'

TOP TIPS

- Make sure that you have enough quality records of evidence for your end-of-rotation reviews to get signed off
- Be honest with your tutors as to whether you should be signed off
- Be prepared for your tutor to ask you to provide more evidence for particular performance standards
- It is not a race to get anywhere first; the number of performance standards that you get signed off at each progress review is irrelevant
- Be confident if you think that you should be signed off
- The end of your life as a pre-reg is just the beginning of your life as a pharmacist

Section 4

Finding your first real job

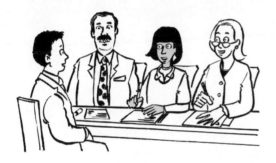

Your first job as a hospital pharmacist

15

FINDING THE RIGHT JOB

It will seem like you have only just got to grips with what pre-registration training entails and suddenly you need to start to think about your first job as a registered pharmacist. There are many issues that you might want to give some thought to, before you even attempt to apply for any jobs:

- Do you want to stay in pharmacy?
- Do you want to stay in hospital or move to community?
- Do you want to get a permanent job or work as a locum?
- Do you want to stay at your current hospital?

It may surprise you but not every pre-reg wants to stay in pharmacy after their pre-reg year; some leave the profession and go off and do something entirely unrelated like asset management whereas others stay in healthcare and go back to university to study medicine, dentistry or do a PhD. Others are sick of 5 years of studying and want to take some time off and go travelling. It is not a given that you will want to stay in pharmacy and whatever you do must be right for you at the time.

The issue of whether you want to stay in hospital pharmacy at all is not discussed in great length within this text because applications and jobs, in industry, community or primary care trusts (PCTs), or continuing your studies further with a PhD is not within the scope of this book.

If you want to stay in pharmacy and in hospital you need to think about which hospital. If you want to stay in your pre-reg hospital, is your hospital used to retaining their pre-regs as qualified pharmacists? If your hospital is not used to this, you may need to think about whether the staff with whom you have been working these past few months are capable of allowing you to make that transition from being a trainee to someone who is qualified. How will the technician who taught you everything that you needed to know about dispensing feel about you being in charge of him or her? There are many pre-regs who would not stay at the hospital as a pharmacist for many different reasons. Obviously, if you did not have a very good time at the hospital where you did your pre-regs, this is an ideal opportunity to make your mark in a different hospital. If you do want to stay at your own hospital, this is obviously a good thing for you because you will know what to expect, or at least have some idea!

'I've only been here a short while but I already know that I am going to move on. No offence to this hospital, it's just that I think that it is best to try to work in as many different places as you can, so that you can learn lots of different things.'

'I would never stay in the hospital where I did my pre-reg year. I think that you'll always get treated like a pre-reg no matter what you do as a pharmacist.'

For some hospitals, especially the larger teaching hospitals, they are used to taking on a certain number of their own pre-regs. This causes other problems, in that your hospital may not be able to take all their own pre-regs. So, you may need to be prepared for rejection from a manager with whom you may still need to work closely, and to carry on working with your fellow pre-reg who HAS got that job. This is the time when you may realise that the pre-reg whom you thought was your close friend very quickly reverts to being someone whom you have known for only a few short months.

Advertisements for hospital jobs as rotational posts appear all year round, but are specifically targeted for pre-registration pharmacists due to qualify that August around January of each year. For NHS hospital jobs the places to look are the *Pharmaceutical Journal*, www.jobs.nhs.uk and www.pjcareers.com. You can subscribe to these websites for email alerts on jobs. If you are thinking of getting a job in a different sector of pharmacy, you obviously have to look elsewhere.

For your first job after pre-registration training, you apply for Band 6 jobs, which are variously advertised as post-registration pharmacists, diploma pharmacists and rotational pharmacists. In terms of rotational jobs, be sure to check that the job really is Band 6 because many hospitals now offer rotational jobs at Band 7, which would not be appropriate for you to apply for.

Although the main responsibilities of these jobs are very similar, there are some details about which you need to find out, to ensure that you really apply for the right job for you. Check your working hours: although most jobs have core contractual hours of 37.5 hours per week, find out how these hours are worked in reality, because it may not be the traditional 9 am–5.30 pm job. Different hospitals operate different working hours, which may include weekend or late-night working. If you are required to work out of hours, you need to clarify what time you get off in lieu, i.e. if you work through a night, what hours do you get back and when are you required to take those hours off?

Be sure to know what the job that you have applied for entails. A residency job is undoubtedly harder work than one that requires an on-call service. Be sure to ask how many other people are on the out-of-hours rota. If you have not checked this out, you may find that you are working every fourth or fifth night if you are unlucky! Doing your homework at this point will pay off, because you don't want to be in a position, after you have accepted a job, of finding out that it is harder work than you envisaged, and impacts on your personal life to a larger degree than you expected.

Find out if the pharmacy service in the hospital to which you are applying sees the out-of-hours service as a continuation of the day service, so that you are providing a full 24-hour pharmacy service, or if it is an emergency service where pharmacy are primarily required to provide advice and only emergency supplies; this makes a massive difference in terms of what you get called for when you are providing out-of-hours service, and will give you a clue as to what is expected from you.

How long you are required to stay in work after hours, and what help you have from any support staff, vary from hospital to hospital, so you need to make sure that you find this out from the department to which you are applying.

Whichever type of job you apply for, at first, you may find it a shock that pharmacy services is solely in your hands, and that you need to make some decisions that, just a few short months before, you were not confident in making!

Be sure to question what type of rotations you have to undertake. It is likely that general medicine and general surgery feature heavily as your major rotations because these general areas contain most of the broad medical and pharmaceutical knowledge base on which to build throughout your career.

Most hospital pharmacy jobs are advertised through websites and you have to fill in online application forms to apply for these jobs, just as with your pre-reg application. As with your pre-reg form, pay attention to what you are writing, because it is likely that the competition for these jobs will be fierce. Copying out what you wrote in your pre-reg application may not be relevant when applying for a pharmacist's job, so be careful!

Most importantly, read the job description, so that you can understand what is required of you in this job, and the person specification, which is the document that sets out what qualities the employer would like from their perfect candidate for the job. The person specification is therefore very useful in terms of formulating your personal statement to support your application. If the person specification tells you exactly what the employer is looking for, make sure that you write about things mentioned. Include examples of work that you have done in your pre-reg that demonstrate that you are the ideal candidate for whom they are looking.

Although you may base this application on your pre-reg application, it is likely that you will need to add a lot more to your statement from the things that you have done as a pre-reg, because many of these things will go a long way to show your prospective employer that you can do the job as a pharmacist.

HOW TO GET THROUGH THE INTERVIEW

Interviews vary in content and length, depending on what employers want from their candidates. Although your prospective employer would like to get to know you, it is also likely that he or she will want to somehow test what you have learnt as a pre-registration trainee pharmacist. This means that you are likely to be presented with some type of sample drug chart with problems that you need to resolve, some calculations and some scenarios that you have to work through. Our main piece of advice is to be yourself as much as possible. Do not try to be someone who you are not because you will be found out – if not at the interview, then when you arrive to start your job.

Answer the interview questions honestly and as fully as you can, without trying to impress your interviewer. Do NOT try to pretend to know what you are talking about when you don't – i.e. guess – because you can guarantee that the person interviewing you knows more that you, especially if you are talking about clinical subjects; the interviewer will have all the experience and expertise and quite probably have had a hand in preparing the sample drug chart that you are being tested on!

Please remember that the whole business of applying for jobs is an incredibly stressful and emotional one, especially when you are in the middle of the pre-reg training year, the most important year of your career so far. Although many pre-regs are ready, willing and able to leap onto that employment treadmill, some want to qualify first and make sure that they can stand on their own two feet by taking locum positions, before applying for any permanent position.

YOUR FIRST JOB

If you had an amazingly supportive pre-registration year, where you were shielded from the realities of the working world, you could find it a total shock when you enter the world of work and earn your keep. You could find that you have very little support from either your supervisors or your line manager, because they are concentrating on service delivery issues rather than making sure that you are ok! The arrangements for who looks after you may also be disorganised because your new place of work expects you to induct yourself into the department to some extent!

You will feel too young and inexperienced to shoulder the massive burden of being a pharmacist. The realities and the responsibilities of being a pharmacist will probably not dawn on you until you have started life as one. As a pre-reg, it would have seemed easy to sign everything that you did, secure in the knowledge that a pharmacist was supervising you and taking responsibility for things that you did on their behalf. As a newly qualified pharmacist, you do not have the luxury of another person taking responsibility for your actions.

You will feel awful the first time that you make a mistake and it will shake your confidence and belief in yourself. But, you must remember that all pharmacists make mistakes in their careers. If every pharmacist who had ever made a mistake stopped being a pharmacist, there would be no pharmacists in the world! People will treat you like a pharmacist even though you may not ever have practised as one.

As you are employed as a pharmacist, many people do not realise that, a few weeks ago, you were 'just a pre-reg'. Many people do not realise that you are carrying out many of your duties for the very first time and that you are relatively inexperienced. In fact, your first year after qualifying as a pharmacist may be harder than your pre-reg year, because not only do you have to learn how to do your job, but you also need to start to take responsibility and be answerable for your actions as well!

You haven't stopped learning. In fact, you will probably learn more in the first 2 years of being a qualified pharmacist than you have learned to date.

You may think that you learned a lot in your pre-registration training year, but the reality is that you learn the most that you may ever learn about being a pharmacist in the first 1–2 years of qualification. There is no substitute for hands-on experience and, within 2 years of qualifying, you are likely to come across the common situations with which you will have to deal for the rest of your career.

Although many of our pre-regs have gone on to fantastic careers in all sectors of pharmacy, there are also many who have made career changes into finance, property management and all sorts. We happily give our blessing to whatever a pre-reg wants to do next, whether in- or outside pharmacy. Whichever direction your decisions take you in is fine, as long as you are happy. And we are sure that, whatever people end up doing, their time as a pre-registration pharmacist has armed them with a raft of invaluable skills that are applicable to many careers and many workplaces.

As this is such a critical step in the process of developing your career, we have included an 'extra' section focusing entirely on more top tips for your interviews. Although you may all be aware of most of these tips, some of them may be useful for you in those stressful moments!

TOP TIPS

- Do your research into the hospitals to which you are likely to apply for a job. Ask the current pre-regs and the current Band 6 pharmacists who work there
- Any information that you want to include in your online application should be put into a Word (or equivalent) document to ensure that any typos or grammatical errors are picked up
- Be aware that your newfound pre-reg friends may not be so friendly if you get the job and they don't
- If your heart is not really in pharmacy, it's ok to make that leap!

ADDITIONAL INTERVIEW TOP TIPS

Preparation for the interview

- Preparation is so important. Make sure that you know a little bit about the job for which you have applied and the organisation into which you entering. Discuss this with someone, because they may be able to help.

- Do some background reading on things that may be relevant to the post for which you are applying. Read the last three or four issues of the *Pharmaceutical Journal* at the very least. Pick out two or three articles and read them thoroughly. Make sure that you have an opinion on your reading and how it is going to influence your practice. Discuss this with someone, remembering to have pros and cons.

- Have two or three interventions that you have made (on the wards, in the dispensary or even in community), and make sure that you are able to discuss them during the interview. It is quite common for these types of questions to be asked.

- If you can, find out if there are any future plans for the department; if you can't find any, make sure that you know about future plans for the NHS. Discuss this with someone so that your opinions are not too extreme – discuss the pros and cons.

Before the interview

- Always arrive at least 30 minutes before your scheduled time for interview (gives you flexibility if you get lost and there is no last-minute panic).

- Go to the loo if you need to as soon as you can.

- Interviews rarely run on time, so use the time you have wisely by looking around the department (you may be able to do this even if you are sitting down somewhere), see if people are talking to each other and if anyone gives you a welcoming look (always a sign of a friendly department).

- Don't do any last-minute reading, because it looks bad and may show lack of preparation. You don't want to start off on the wrong foot!

- Make sure that you either have a drink of water or chew some gum (but remember to get rid of it) as you want to keep your mouth moist. It is amazing how quickly your mouth dries out when you are nervous in an interview. If this happens to you take your drink in with you. In some interviews they provide you with water but not always.

- Make sure that you look presentable and confident; give them the impression that they need you more than you need them.

- If you can start talking to someone, it will help calm your nerves and also pass the time.

- If you are going on a tour of the department ask lots of questions about the people and the set-up. Ask about your potential role. Have a look at the people working: are they talking to each other, are there any smiling faces, do people give you welcoming looks or are they too busy? Who is showing you around? Make sure that you look and sound interested.

During the interview

- Relax and be confident. More importantly, be yourself because this is who we want to see!
- Relax but also keep your guard up at all times.
- **First impressions are crucial; from the moment someone calls you for your turn, the interview has started. Smile!**
- When you enter the room look at everyone. Sometimes the interviewers will stand up and introduce themselves; look at each one, smile and say something (hello, hi). Wait for them to put their hand out to shake (some may do this, some may not). Look at each person individually and wait for him or her to ask you to sit down.
- You will be nervous now and we expect this, so the leader of the interview will explain the format and ask you some easy questions about yourself. (Why did you chose this job? Describe how you have got here. Describe your career history.) We may have the answers on your application form so make sure that you say the same things as you wrote there.
- The key thing is to relax and be yourself.
- The interviewers usually take it in turns to ask questions; make sure that you look at everyone when answering but focus on the questioner. Be careful with eye contact; it is not essential to maintain eye contact if it makes you uncomfortable. If you need to think, look away and regain eye contact when you answer.
- There may be some hard questions for which you have not prepared. Don't worry; take your time in answering the question. If you don't understand the question then ask for it to be **rephrased**. Ensure that you understand the question before you start to answer it. Remember that this is not an exam; it is a two-way process. If you forget the question or think that you have missed the point, ask the interviewer if you have answered the question. A good interviewer will usually prompt you at this stage.
- Don't worry if you don't know the answer to a knowledge question; don't panic and say that you have not come across this before

(unless you genuinely haven't; these questions are usually targeted at your level). If it is a clinical question think logically and start from basics. The main thing is not to guess; if you don't know, say so.

- Try to talk as much as you can although don't overdo it. It is easy to start repeating yourself; once you have said all you can, stop.

- You don't need to answer a question straightaway; sometimes it may be better to think about things for a minute or two before you answer.

- The questions are usually based on the job description and person's specification from the post and there should be few surprises. They are generally split into:

  - questions about you
  - questions specific to the post
  - questions showing evidence of background reading.

- After we have finished interviewing you, we give you the opportunity to ask us some questions. Make sure that you have two or three questions (sometimes you may not have any or your questions may be answered during the interview). If you do not have any questions then say that all your questions were answered during the interview (we won't know what your questions were anyway).

- Make sure that your questions are good in that they are relevant. Usually they can be about start dates or accommodation should you need it.

- Don't ask about money because you can get that information elsewhere. One good question that we have been asked is: 'You have heard what I can do for you. What can you do for me or what are you able to offer me?' A bit brave but a good question nevertheless.

- It may be an idea to discuss your questions with someone; if you are prone to forgetting them then write them down. We don't mind this as long as it is not a long list of questions about which you should have found out yourself.

- At the end of the interview we go through some housekeeping for personnel. This is routine and not really part of the 'interview' but the interview is still not over. We may ask you about contacting your referee, so it is important that your referee knows about your interview. We also ask you for a contact number; if you have a mobile then know the number. If this is what you give us, then remember to keep it on and the battery charged, because we may need to contact you quite soon after the interview. Decisions can be made very quickly!

- When the interview is finished make sure that you thank everyone for his or her time. It is a nice touch. Some people shake hands at the end, others don't. Wait and see what the response is from the interviewers.
- The interview is not over until you have left the department so maintain your composure until you are out of sight. You don't know what the competition is like and you may have a good chance, so don't blow it at the end.

After the interview

- The panel usually inform you when they will be getting in touch. If you have not heard from them in that time then get in touch yourself. We do not normally contact everyone and you may not be contacted because you may be second on the list and we need to wait for confirmation from our number one choice (people do change their minds and refuse jobs).
- At this point you need to make your mind up if this is the job that you want because your mind may have been changed at the interview. Under no circumstances should you accept straightaway unless you are 100% sure. Take at least a night to think things over; discuss it with someone.
- If you do accept the job, it is offered pending appropriate references and occupational health clearance. This is standard practice. Accept the job and say that it depends on having the offer confirmed in writing. Again this is normal practice.
- If you have another interview you must be clear with them. Don't accept a job and then change your mind. It is better to say that you cannot accept it until you have had the other interview. If we want you, we can wait for you. You have to be open about this because, if you refuse, we can at least offer it to someone else. It would be worth discussing this with someone as well.
- If you do not get the job, ask for specific feedback on your performance. This is so that you can improve for next time. Good interviewers are normally only too happy to do this.

Section 5

Preparing for the registration exam

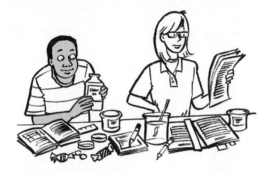

16

Preparing for the registration exam

HOW MUCH TO REVISE, WHEN TO REVISE, WHAT TO REVISE?

The issue of what to revise is a tricky one because the Royal Pharmaceutical Society of Great Britain (RPSGB) registration examination is unlike any other exams that you have done before. So, what to revise then?

If you ask your colleagues, each person will tell you something different to revise, so all we can do is give you some suggestions, hints, tips, dos and don'ts, but you need to make your own judgement on what works best for you.

You probably won't start to think about the exam until about your 39-week Progress Report 3. This is because, at this report, your tutor discusses your progress to date with you and whether you can attain the remainder of the performance standards to become competent, and feel able to take the registration examination, so you can then be entered for the examination at that point.

The first thing to do is to look at the exam syllabus, which is contained within your RPSGB pre-reg training manual (if you haven't been referring to this throughout your training year that is!). This gives you some pointers as to the subject areas that you need to cover. It is very clear that the registration examination is not so much about cramming knowledge into your brain, but being able to analyse and evaluate practice-based problems. This indicates that you should have learned most of your knowledge from your everyday practice at work. The exam syllabus is not laid out in detail. You do not need in-depth knowledge of all the syllabus topic areas to answer questions in the closed book paper, because a pharmacist in practice would refer to information sources for more in-depth knowledge. What you DO need is to have a good working knowledge of the basic and common aspects of pharmacy that come up in practice.

So, in reality, you have been preparing for your registration exam since the day that you started your pre-registration training!

REFERENCE TEXTS

The reference texts for the open book examination are the obvious place to start as useful revision tools, but they are not the only ways in which you might like to prepare for the registration examination. You may need to invest in a good pharmacology and therapeutics book, which should give you some good background into the pathology of the conditions that you come across, because it is unlikely that the *British National Formulary* (BNF) has much information on this.

British National Formulary

Some people may suggest that you read the *BNF* from cover to cover. We are not so sure how useful this is. It is not a novel, so it doesn't read very well. The monographs are also pretty much just a list of various facts about each drug, so how you are supposed to remember any of this just by reading through is beyond us. What you need to do is use everyday triggers to direct you to what you look up.

In your everyday practice, you handle drugs or drug-related issues, so what you need to do is to keep looking at your *BNF* every time that you come across something that you do not know. When you have looked at the same page for the hundredth time you might remember what was on that page!

It is very difficult to revise from the monographs, because they are basically just lists of unconnected words that are hard to remember. Do read the introductions to drugs for broad overviews of each topic areas. Use everyday triggers (e.g. MI enquiries, discharge prescriptions [TTOs]) to encourage revision rather than reading blindly. *Remember that everything in the texts is examinable including information on the covers!* Make a list of items that you commonly encounter in practice, e.g. antibiotics, cardiac medicines, respiratory medicines, diabetes medicines, pain relievers, thera-peutic drug monitoring (TDM) and enzyme inducers/inhibitors. Try to think what in your everyday practice is most likely to be examined. Throughout the text there are many warnings from the Commission on Human Medicines (CHM, formerly the CSM or Commission on the Safety of Medicines); make a note of all of these because it is important information.

'I had a stress attack 2 weeks ago. I didn't know how to start going through the *BNF*. I'm not a person who can leave it until the end so I'm doing a little bit every day, otherwise I'll panic if I leave it too late. It is difficult to deal with other people's stresses about the exam though and keep focused on me.'

Medicines, Ethics and Practice Guide

Unfortunately there is no substitute for reading the *Medicines, Ethics and Practice* (MEP) guide (RPSGB). At least it is written in sentences. One thing to say would be that it is not particularly well indexed so you may need to make your own, more detailed index. Also, remember to cross-reference all the information that can also be found in the BNF – the information for some of the exam questions may be found in more than one text so you need to work out which text contains that most complete information and also which text you prefer to work with.

Drug Tariff

The *Drug Tariff* is another text that is incredibly hard to read, because it is not designed to be read from cover to cover, but as a reference source for pricing issues. It may be useful to refer to the *NPA Guide to the Drug Tariff*, which takes you section by section through the *Drug Tariff*. In the registration exam, there is usually a question about prescription charges and pharmacist professional fees, so this section is obviously an important section to look at.

Remember, however, that much of your learning will not be from revising but from your everyday practice. Do not go through the pre-reg year blindly; pay attention to the patients whom you see and the drugs that you come into contact with, because you are likely to remember things better if you have encountered them in your everyday practice.

HOW WILL YOU FEEL LEADING UP TO THE EXAM?

'I feel fine. I still need to sort out my *Drug Tariff* and questions but I'm not too worried about it. I still want to know a bit more about CSM warnings. I'm using some of my study time in my dispensary rotation to do some revision. For me, essay writing is ok but MCQ questions are a nightmare, so I'm going to need to develop some strategies.'

'I have been considering not sitting the exam. I look at others and think that they know so much more than me. I'm not just worried about the exam but also about being competent as a pharmacist. I'm not confident at the moment that I can pass the exam and be a good pharmacist, which is what I have always wanted to do'

'I'm happy about being entered in for the exam. I haven't started doing calculations properly yet and I've not started doing exam revision yet either. I plan to start sometime in May.'

'I think it will be fine to pass the exam. No problems. I'm more concerned about being competent. I have always been good at passing exams so I won't get stressed out. I'm not planning to book holiday to prepare for it.'

After having done a full-day mock exam, the issues below are the ones that were highlighted for some pre-regs.

Closed Book

- Many pre-regs felt unhappy and that they knew nothing.
- But there's plenty time, because you either do or don't know it.

Exam technique

- Review your answers BUT go with first 'gut' instincts – you have a feeling for a particular answer probably because you have seen it before; try NOT to change all your initial answers.

Practicalities

- Thirst: take in bottled water. Make sure that you drink – but not too much! And always go to the loo before entering the exam hall.
- Bring layers of clothing – you have no idea how hot or cold the exam hall is going to be.
- Remember to bring a spare pencil/sharpener/rubber.

Security issues

- Make sure that you know where your texts are during the closed book exam. Keep them safe so that you can use them in the afternoon.

Open book/calculations

- Some pre-regs felt much less happy than with the closed book!
- Some felt very tired due to it being after lunch!

Exam technique

- RAN OUT OF TIME! No one left early.
- Do calcs first (if that's how you want to do it).
- Calculations ran over so less time for the open book questions.
- Did not plan time well enough.
- Unwilling to move on from a question that didn't know how to do, so lost time.
- Some things you DON'T NEED TO LOOK UP – YOU KNOW THEM ALREADY!
- Write your reference page number on your exam paper – you may need to refer to the same page later on in the exam.
- Fold/mark pages/bookmark with pencils and rubbers etc. to bookmark pages if referring to multiple pages for a question.
- When you find the right answer – STOP LOOKING!
- NEVER LEAVE A BLANK ANSWER FOR A QUESTION – when time is called for 5 minutes till the end – GUESS ANYTHING YOU DON'T KNOW.

Practicalities

- Where are you going to keep your books? May not be enough space on your desk – lap?
- If you are susceptible to distraction from noises (hundreds of pages turning!) take earplugs into the exam hall.
- Energy levels may dip in the middle of the exam – have sugary drinks/ snacks at the ready.
- Do not bring in NOISY food.

Revision plans

After the mock exam, many pre-regs felt that they:

- did not know references well enough;
- did not know *Drug Tariff* and *MEP Guide*.

DRAWING FROM PAST PRE-REGS' EXPERIENCES

Ask your newly qualified pharmacists how they prepared for their registration examination. But remember to get a range of different advice from different people, because you need to find what works for you.

CALCULATIONS AND THE ANXIETIES ASSOCIATED WITH THIS

Calculations are the biggest worry for most pre-regs. The thought of doing calculations without a calculator under exam pressure is a daunting prospect, and the worry stems from the fact that you MUST pass the calculations section of the open book exam at 70% otherwise you will fail. This is partly dealt with by the RPSGB stating that you must not be entered for the registration examination unless you are consistently passing maths tests at 80%, thereby giving you an allowance of a 10% drop in performance during the actual examination.

There are several pharmaceutical calculations books that you should purchase if you are particularly worried.

One thing to say about the calculations in the examination paper is that there will be a lot of what we call 'window dressing', where the question seems to be dressed up in a scenario that you may have never been in before and the question is about a drug that you have never come across before. But the thing to remember is that none of the above matters. What matters is what the question is asking you and sometimes that can be hard to figure out as you may get bamboozled by the myriad of numbers that the question throws at you.

'I feel all right about the exam. Calculations are a bit more sorted. I know that if I overdo it will get bored. I got myself a calculations book. I feel like the closed book questions are ok; I'm happy with them.'

'I'm scared about the exam but will obviously be fine. I'm confident in calculations; in fact, I'm bored of calculations now. I am happy overall with all the past papers that I've done. I've started doing some revision and have got some exam practice. I'm not going to get stressed out because in my rotation I am not around everyone at the moment.'

'I have been doing some calculations practice. It is good to do the mock to see your baseline. Most of the questions can be answered based on what I have learnt already.'

SOME TOP TIPS FOR CALCULATIONS

● Know the different types of pharmaceutical calculations that you might get – from dilutions to ratios. Use basic pharmaceutical calculation books to work through each different type of question to find out which calculations you can do well and, more importantly, identify your weaknesses and practise these types of questions.

- Use past papers to practise but remember that any past paper questions could contain out-of-date information.
- When revising, don't peak too soon: pace your revision. One analogy that we use again and again is to say that athletes do not train for their events months before they are going to compete. Training starts relatively near the event, and escalates in frequency and intensity the nearer the event is. Do not peak too soon by doing questions and papers months in advance of the examination; you will probably get bored and, more importantly, you will run out of fresh resources to work with when you most need them.
- Be careful with units and know unit conversions: always unify your units otherwise the answer that you get may be confusing.
- Remember to simplify your numbers down where possible (i.e. divide all your numbers down with a common denominator so that you have the smallest numbers to work with) and avoid long multiplication/ division to avoid mistakes, unless you are very confident about your long multiplication/division skills under intense examination pressure. Under pressure, it is very easy to forget to carry over your '1s' or to misplace a decimal point!
- The rule of thumb is that most calculations will require you to work in multiples of 2, 5, 10 and 7.
- Consider what a reasonable answer is, and eliminate obviously wrong answers from the selection early on. This means that you will have fewer alternatives to choose from as your final answer.
- Remember that the calculation questions are part of the open book paper, which means that you may need to find some supplementary information to your questions from your reference texts.
- For each calculation question, decide what information is relevant and ignore all the 'window dressing'.
- Try to overcome exam pressure by doing the calculations first in the open book examination.
- Above all, remember that you can get six wrong in the registration examination and still pass!

THE EXAMINATION

The registration examination consists of two papers:

1. In the morning you sit a closed book paper lasting 1.5 hours. This is 90 minutes for 90 questions, which means that you have 1 minute per question.

2.   In the afternoon you sit the open book paper. This lasts for 2.5 hours (150 minutes). The paper is in two parts, with 70 open book questions and 20 calculation questions at the back.

The RPSGB suggest that you split your time up in the following way.

Calculations

•   20 questions to do in 1 hour, which works out at around 3 minutes per calculation question.

Open book questions

•   70 questions to do in $1^1/_2$ hours (90 minutes), which means that each question should take you just over 1 minute.

There are several different question types of which the simplest is:

'Each of the questions or incomplete statements in this section is followed by five suggested answers. Select the best answer in each case.'

This means that you must pick the correct answer out of a list of five possible answers. This is the simplest and most straightforward question that will appear in any of the papers.

'For each numbered question select from the list above it the one lettered option which is most closely related to it. Within each group of questions each lettered option may be used once, more than once or not at all.'

This means that you are presented with a list of five possible solutions. Then you get a number of questions where the answer is one of those five possible answers. As it says, each possible answer may be used once, more than once or not at all.

'Each of the questions or incomplete statements in this section is followed by three responses. For each question ONE or MORE of the responses is (are) correct. Decide which of the responses is (are) correct. Then choose:

A   If 1, 2 and 3 are correct
B   If 1 and 2 only are correct
C   If 2 and 3 only are correct
D   If 1 only is correct
E   If 3 only is correct.'

This type of question is more complicated, and it is likely that the solution to any of these questions comes in several different stages, meaning that you have to find out, work out or calculate several different things for just one mark.

'The following questions consist of a statement in the left-hand column followed by a second statement in the right hand column. Decide whether the first statement is true or false. Decide whether the second statement is true or false. Then choose:

A   If both statements are true and the second statement is a correct explanation of the first statement
B   If both statements are true but the second statement is NOT a correct explanation of the first statement
C   If the first statement is true but the second statement is false
D   If the first statement is false but the second statement is true
E   If both statements are false.'

Many people get very confused with this type of question. Once again, it is likely that the solution to any of these questions comes in several different stages, meaning that you will have to find out, work out or calculate several different things for just one mark. The difference here is the LINK between the different parts of the answer. The best way to link the parts together is by putting the word 'BECAUSE' between your two statements. If STATEMENT 1 happens 'BECAUSE' of STATEMENT 2 then you can be confident that there is a link between the two statements. If putting 'BECAUSE' between the two statements doesn't make sense, then there is unlikely to be a connection between the two statements even if both statements are true.

Generally, the simpler types of questions appear at the beginning of the paper. This holds true for both papers, including the calculation questions. This may dictate for you in which order you should tackle the papers.

PERMITTED REASONABLE ADJUSTMENTS

The RPSGB can accommodate candidates who may require some adjustments because of disability or impairment to allow them a fair go at the exam. Discuss this with your tutor fairly early on if you need such adjustments. You then have to submit a request to the RPSGB stating what you need and why you need it, together with appropriate evidence such as a medical report or letter. As only a small number of candidates need adjustments, you may have to take your exam in an exam centre that can accommodate these adjustments, which may not be the exam centre where your colleagues take theirs. Further information can be obtained from the RPSGB.

IF YOU ARE NOT READY – DO NOT SIT IT; THREE STRIKES AND YOU'RE OUT!

If you are not 100% sure that you are ready for the registration examination, then DO NOT SIT IT. If you really are not sure, there is no point in wasting one of your three chances at passing the examination. It really is three strikes and you're out!

The only requirements about sitting your first attempt at the registration examination are that you must sit it within a certain timeframe after completion of your pre-registration training. Please refer to the RPSGB pre-reg training manual for up-to-date details.

We regularly get pre-regs asking us what we would say if they told us that they did not want to take the exam, and our response is to say that we would shake their hand. It would be a brave decision for any pre-reg to pull out of taking the registration exam; any such decision should be highly respected and supported by tutors.

WHAT HAPPENS IF YOU FAIL?

If you fail your first attempt at the registration examination, you will receive information from the RPSGB that includes a breakdown of your marks. You will also get information on how to enter for the next sitting of the registration examination. Between your first and second attempts, there is no requirement that you undertake any further training, but it might be a good idea to do so just to keep your mind in 'pharmacy' mode. If you fail the registration examination at your second attempt, you need to undertake a further period of pre-registration training, which is normally for a minimum period of 6 months, before you can re-sit it for the third and final time.

If you have failed, you need to be very focused in terms of rectifying the issues that might have let you down on your previous attempt at the registration examination. Talk to your fellow pre-regs and find out what they might have done that helped them to pass. Speak to your tutor to get their view on why you didn't do so well.

There are many different reasons why pre-regs fail the registration examination, some of which are listed below.

Illness/circumstances impairing your ability to sit the examination

You might have been very well prepared but did not feel very well on the day, or there may have been some things happening in your personal life that made you not perform well on the day, such as a close family bereavement, relationship breakdown, sudden onset of illness, etc. The RPSGB has procedures to deal with pre-regs who think that they performed poorly in their registration examination. You can do one of several things:

- You can withdraw before or on the day of the examination. This means that this attempt will not be counted and you can be treated as though you have not made an entry.
- If you are taken ill during the registration examination OR you have been ill leading up to the registration examination and decide to go ahead and sit the exam, but feel that you have been affected adversely by your illness, you can:
  - request to be granted a pass; this can happen only if you believe that you have only narrowly missed the pass mark
  - request to have the examination attempt nullified; if you think that you did REALLY badly because of undue circumstances, you will be treated as if you never took the registration exam at that attempt.

Be careful though; if you are not sure that you are fit (or well prepared enough) to sit the exam, decide to do so, and then 'wait and see' whether you do ok, and then decide to appeal, this will NOT be viewed favourably by the Society. If you KNOW that you are not well or that there are circumstances that will affect your performance, then you MUST report this beforehand. In real life, as a pharmacist, you always need to make a personal judgement as to whether you are fit to work. If you are NOT, YOU are responsible for informing people and removing yourself from situations that may endanger patients' wellbeing. The principles are the same for the registration examination.

Up-to-date information, including the procedures that you need to follow, can be found in your pre-reg training manual or online at www.rpsgb.org. uk. Please refer to this documentation before you proceed with any action.

Calculations

It is easy to feel under pressure about doing calculations in an exam setting. This is why the RPSGB requires you to be able to comfortably get 80% in calculations, to allow for a 10% drop in performance during your exam. Being confident about your calculation skills seems to be the key here. If you are unsure of what you are doing, even if you are right, you are likely to revise some answers that are correct.

Poor exam technique

Generally, candidates find the closed book paper in the morning achievable in the 1.5 hours allocated. This is because, with this paper, you either know it, or you don't, or to some extent you can work it out and make an educated guess.

Many candidates find the open book paper the much harder paper to sit. This is despite (or maybe because of!) the fact that you should have all the answers at your fingertips. The reality is that it is difficult and time-consuming to navigate though the texts. In addition to this, the examination hall tables may not be big enough to accommodate the texts to which you have to refer.

EXPERIENCES FROM OUR PRE-REGS: HOW DID THEY FEEL, WHAT WERE THEIR CONCERNS?

'I was seriously bricking it before the exam. I had taken 5 days off to revise but to be honest, I probably didn't need it although it made me feel better as I felt that if I needed time I had it. I didn't read any text in full and I think tagging my references and knowing where to find things quickly was the most helpful thing. Other than that, most of my exam revision was doing past papers. I also tried to read all of the CSM warnings in the BNF but to be honest I am not sure how helpful it was. I felt that the actual exam was OK. The morning part had gone quite well. During lunchtime it was nice to meet up with other people as the time went quicker and we had already agreed not to talk about the exam. After the exam, I was relieved that it was all over and fairly happy with how it went. I tried not to think about it but blatantly went and looked up all the answers later on.'

'In terms of last minute revision, I did lots of papers and this is the best way to revise. I did BNF quizzes that were given to us at study days and other ones devised by tutors. I used those MCQ books in pharmacy (borrowed from the library); some of the questions were good, others out of date. I had access to a CD-ROM. I used the CD on days I was tired as it was a change from reading and more interactive. I learned the inhibitors and inducers. I did lots of calculations. I listed all the CHM warnings and advice in the BNF (I filled in what they were and what page in the BNF they were on; I used this to tag my BNF). I also listed all the hepatotoxic drugs, drugs that cause blood dyscrasias, a list of drugs that need counselling (I filled in what the counselling points were), and drugs with warning cards, etc. In fact this document was a useful summary of important sections in the BNF. I tagged everything in the MEP and just bits of the *Drug Tariff*. I found the mock exams very helpful for timing purposes.'

'I remember on the morning of the exam we all gathered together and walked to the exam together. I remember there was lots of last minute cramming just before the exam and we had lists of things like name all the drugs that cause metallic taste and then someone would read out the answer as we were all trying to think what they were. I didn't think this stressful but if you did, there were other people talking about their plans for the summer party/ball and the night out that was ahead of us. I remember there were friends of mine doing the exam from uni and I had arranged to meet up with them before the exam to say good luck.'

'I got a bit nervous about finding my room and the invigilator was very strict about what you could have on the desk (so I don't think you could have lucky mascots which might be a shock to some people); he also got cross if you spoke to anybody. The room was very crowded and there is not much space between candidates.'

'During the exam it's all very industrious. I do remember having enough time for the closed book, our first exam – I felt this was a bit easier then the open book exam. I ran out of time on the open book. I did my calculations first – I thought they were really difficult in the exam and went over the time (by about 5 minutes on them). I did complete them though before I moved on. I guessed the last two or three questions in the exam (educated guesses though). The thing to remember in the exam is to watch the time and do the calculations first and everything else follows.'

'Afterwards I met a friend from uni and we discussed the exam and both convinced ourselves we had failed. I only remembered the questions I had problems with and she did as well. In reality I was happy it was over and had a great night out afterwards. I really was not too worried if I had to re-sit as I had all the info; it was just a case of knowing it a bit better. I passed the exam and really did not believe it! I was thrilled.'

TOP TIPS

- Have a go at doing the open book backwards
- Open book: calculations 3 min/question; open slightly more than 1 min/question – MAKE SURE THAT YOU DON'T EXCEED 1 HOUR ON CALCULATIONS
- If you know an open answer question, stop looking up!
- Write the page number of the reference that you have used for each question down, so that, if you need that same reference further in the paper, you know exactly where to go
- Make sure that you mark the correct answer box: use a long ruler if helpful
- In the open book, the answers ALWAYS come from the text, i.e. it is possible that the same question has different answers across the two papers in areas where there have been very recent changes, e.g. CDs, pseudoephedrine; therefore in the open book always check the references
- Don't leave any empty spaces; there is no negative marking so guessing is encouraged
- In the closed book, if you don't know an answer then move on
- Remember that you have to get 70% to pass, i.e. you can get 30% of questions wrong and still pass!

REFERENCES

NHS England and Wales. *Drug Tariff*. London: The Stationery Office, published monthly.

Joint Formulary Committee. *British National Formulary*. London: British Medical Association and Royal Pharmaceutical Society of Great Britain, published six-monthly.

RPSGB. *Medicines, Ethics and Practice: A guide for pharmacists and pharmacy technicians*. London: Royal Pharmaceutical Society of Great Britain, published annually.

The NPA Guide to the Drug Tariff and NHS Dispensing for England and Wales. National Pharmaceutical Association, 2002.

Section 6

Specialist placements

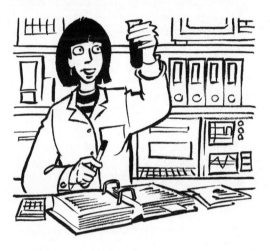

Integrated sandwich courses

17

At the time of writing, there is currently just one university that offers a sandwich course programme for pharmacy, which includes two periods of 6 months in the workplace undertaking pre-registration training. These sandwich courses are not truly integrated in terms of how the planned integration of pre-registration training into the undergraduate programme will happen over the next few years.

The Bradford University programme involves two placements: the first in the second 6 months of the third year and the second in the first 6 months of the fifth year. It is recommended to students that one placement be undertaken in the community sector and the other in the hospital, although this is not always possible because it depends on the placements being available. In terms of a traditional pre-reg year, the first placement is seen as the fifth year placement because it takes place in the first 6 months of the pre-reg year, and the second placement as the third year placement because it is in the second 6 months.

Undertaking either of your placements in hospital pharmacy can be beneficial and detrimental in different ways, which we explore here.

FIRST PLACEMENT – FIFTH YEAR (JULY TO JANUARY)

The first, and probably the most important, thing to say about the fifth year placement is that this is actually the second 6 months of pre-registration training. You need to settle in quicker and be more focused on achieving all that is required to be signed off as competent at the end of your placement than your contemporaries. If you have done your first placement in community pharmacy you will inevitably be using this as your benchmark for practice. Be warned that hospital pharmacy can be very different and the roles and responsibilities of the staff around you may also be very different. You will be working with a wider range of pharmacy support staff in the hospital, some of whom have quite senior roles that may be more senior than some pharmacists.

There is an expectation that you have done 6 months of pre-registration training, so you know what is required in terms of demonstrating your competence and completing records of evidence. In community pharmacy you work alongside your tutor and therefore are under constant observation, so your tutor may not require so many records of evidence because he or she will have seen you practising. As discussed before, this may not be the case in hospital where you may never work alongside your tutor.

The range of work encountered in community pharmacy is quite narrow compared with what you encounter in the hospital. Although you may encounter clinical activities in the community such as medicines use reviews, minor ailment schemes and community-based clinics such as anti-coagulation clinics, most of the bread-and-butter work in the community is still dispensing prescriptions and providing over-the-counter advice for common and minor ailments. It is not uncommon to see pre-regs who have completed their first 6 months coming to hospital with most of the performance standards signed off. This can sometimes show a lack of understanding of the nature of a sandwich course placement, because it is unlikely that you will be competent to practise at the end of the third year of your degree programme. Many tutors will want to go through your portfolio of evidence and review your records of evidence for themselves; some tutors may even go further and ask you to review what you were signed off for at the end of the first placement and think whether you really are competent. Remember that the tutor in the second placement holds the ultimate responsibility of signing you off.

In the hospital, you need to demonstrate competence in dispensing, clinical ward-based pharmacy, medicines information and some form of manufacturing (sterile, non-sterile, aseptic), which presents a serious challenge of settling in quickly and working to a high enough level in each of the rotations.

Pre-regs have in the past thought that they were nearly there when they arrived but after seeing what was required have re-thought how close they are to being a pharmacist. When asked to give a number out of 10 for where they thought they were, the average number was between 2 and 3. These pre-regs had obviously recognised how much work still needed to be done; one pre-reg even went so far as to say that he would give himself only 9 out of 10 after 10 years of practice. This highlights how different pre-regs see the roles and responsibilities of a pharmacist.

The unique aspects of the sandwich programme are that, as you have completed your first placement, you already come with some transferable skills in terms of being able to work quickly and accurately while under pressure, and being able to prioritise work and communicate with patients and doctors. The year back at university then builds on your pre-registration experience and increases your knowledge, making it more relevant to the patient. This is something that a traditional 12-month pre-reg still has to learn.

Another difficult situation is that, even though you have completed 6 months of pre-reg training, you may still lack clinical knowledge. This is because, in the current set-up, medicines management modules start in the fourth year and are not examined until the end of the fifth year, which means that, even though you may have developed skills in terms of being a professional pharmacist at an early stage, you may still lack confidence when compared with a traditional 12-month pre-reg at the start of your pre-reg because the latter has completed all his or her degree programme. That said, exposure to real patients and clinical problems means that you can relate to these better in lectures and in exams. You may be lucky enough to see a patient with a rash as an adverse drug reaction, which appears in one of your examinations.

In the hospital, depending on the structure of your programme, you get only one shot at each rotation because there is probably not enough time to go back and revisit a rotation. Some hospitals provide you with a wide range of short rotations where you see lots of areas of hospital practice, whereas others limit the range of rotations to allow you enough time to consolidate your learning into practice. It can sometimes be difficult for staff training you to understand your specific needs because they may put you in the bracket of a traditional 12-month pre-reg and have lower expectations of you. It is up to you to remind them that you are a 6-month pre-reg, and completing your training in 6 months, and therefore you need to be ready to be signed off. It is up to you to drive your own training, which many pre-regs have found difficult initially – how do you inform someone whom you hardly know that they are not training you sufficiently when you cannot do what is being asked of you to the level required? You need to take time to adjust to new ways of working but the difficulty is you yourself recognising when to push your progress or sit back a little and consolidate. Your tutor should be able to guide you because he or she has an idea of what is required and what is yet to come.

Your formal progress review around October, 39 weeks, is the time when the rest of the pre-regs undergo their 13-week progress reviews. Although the focus for the rest of the pre-regs is on how they have settled into working and not being a student, you are discussing how close you are to being a pharmacist and what performance standards you need to focus on in the remaining time that you have. This adds to the pressure so you need to be more organised than your colleagues and more focused at an early stage. Your next progress review generally takes place in the New Year and you should be ready at this stage to be signed off. The difference for you is that sitting the registration exam and being a pharmacist are still some time away because you have to return to university and complete the last term and your final exams and assignments. You need to be careful that you don't slip back into the old habits of being a student.

SECOND PLACEMENT – THIRD YEAR (JANUARY TO JULY)

The biggest issue for this placement is settling in and integrating into an existing pre-reg team. This can be very difficult, particularly if the team is large and settled into well-established roles and hierarchies. The fact that, as a third year, you are a few years younger than your colleagues, have little or no real pharmacy experience and may not have the confidence to integrate into the team can make the placement really difficult.

Recruiting third year placement students is often the most difficult thing to do because these students can have very limited experience and there is a large element of taking a risk or going on a hunch in terms of whether they would fit into the workplace. It is really up to you how you approach the placement; you can either focus on getting the work done and approach everything from an academic point of view, calling each rotation a module, or focus more on getting to know the people around you, what they do and how they got to where they are. Fitting in socially is an important element of this placement because, depending on where you go, you may end up living away from the family home far away from your family and usual circle of friends. In our experience, this can be the most daunting part of the programme and it can take some time for you to actually feel that you belong.

Another aspect that is really important is that you are coming into the second half of the year where the other pre-regs around you are focusing initially on getting their next jobs as a pharmacist, then worrying about being signed off at the end of the year, while having the registration exam at the back of their minds. For you, none of these things is important because you are still a few years away from this. Some of you may choose to keep out of these aspects and concentrate on your own training whereas others feel that to belong in the team they would prefer to join and learn from what is going on around them. Note that when it is your turn to look for jobs and prepare for the registration exam, you will be back at university and will not have such a support network of peers to lean on.

In terms of the actual work that you need to be doing, you are paid the same amount of money as the rest of the pre-regs but can't perform at their level. Many of the training staff around you won't know what is meant by the Bradford University sandwich course or not treat you any differently from the other pre-regs. This may particularly be the case if you are in a rotation alongside a traditional 12-month pre-reg. This can sometimes be a good thing because it informs you about the level of practice that you should be at, although it can also cause you to worry that you will never attain their level and that you may be letting the people around you down because you just don't have the experience. If you feel like this you should try to explain to your supervisor how your course works and what you have, and have not, done at university so far. There will inevitably be large gaps in your knowledge where you have not covered certain topics in your course, but you cannot always use this as an excuse. For hospitals that take Bradford University students, the tutors know what you have and have not covered because the University sends a copy of the degree programme to the tutors. Although sometimes it can be appropriate to say that you are a Bradford third year when you do not know something, you cannot always hide behind this!

In terms of each rotation that you encounter, you may not have done any dispensary work in your life other than pharmacy practice classes at university, which do not really replicate the experience of real-life work because you are never under that same pressure in a classroom. It may be that you only just learn how to label and accurately dispense prescriptions in your dispensary rotation. Do not compare what you are doing with what the other pre-regs are doing because they are looking to be signed off as competent in the second half of their year and you are not. There can be a tendency for you to want to do whatever they are doing in terms of clinically screening prescriptions and undertaking patient counselling. Remember that these activities require application of some clinical knowledge and experience, both of which are not available at this stage of your career.

For ward-based clinical pharmacy rotations, you should be able to undertake medication histories by asking patients about their medications because the initial part of a medication history is essentially a technical process. Once you have learned how to take a medication history and know what questions you need to ask, try turning this into a conversation with the patient rather than obviously going through a checklist. It may take you some time to build your confidence and experience before you really feel comfortable in doing this. There will be lots of times when you record drugs that you have never heard of and consequently know nothing about. It is these drugs that you want to list for further reading in terms of their mechanisms of action and their place in therapy for your patients. You can then work out whether these drugs should be on the drug chart or whether they were intentionally left off.

For medicines information, the biggest problem for you is linked to having no idea what the drugs are, because, once you have gone through the initial training workbook and have progressed to answering the phones, you may not know which questions to ask that would be relevant for the drug in question. Either you may ask all the questions and risk asking questions that are not relevant to the problem, but you won't know this, or in a panic you do not ask the right questions at all! Your supervising pharmacist can guide you and there may be occasions when you either have to ring the enquirer back or have to pass the phone on to someone else because you are completely out of your depth. Remember that this may not be a reflection on you, just that people are contacting medicines information because they have a question themselves and do not know the answer. You may be able to take down the enquiry and have a think about what the real question is before starting a search strategy. You should keep your supervising pharmacist involved at all times until they allow you more scope to work on your answer before discussing it with them.

Production, or manufacturing, should be no different for you compared with the other pre-regs because you all enter the rotation with the same knowledge base, generally zero.

While this may all sound very challenging, there is a lot to be said for having this experience at such an early stage of your career and degree programme. It means that you are more able to put your lectures at university into context because you may have seen patients with some of the disease conditions being discussed in lectures in real life. You may even be in a position to inform your lecturers that what it says in their lectures and what it says in textbooks are not what happens in real life, and that practice has moved ahead! Not all of you will be brave enough to say anything!

Last, in terms of performance standards, do not expect to be signed off for so many. As you will undertake a further 6-month placement in a year's time, many of the performance standards need to be reassessed and signed off by the second pre-reg tutor. Ask any traditional 12-month pre-reg and you will be told that things tend to fall into place in the second half of the year and, for you, that second half has yet to come.

The whole experience can be summed up by this quote from a sandwich course student.

'I initially applied for the 5-year course to get experience in both hospital and community (pharmacy) because I had very little pharmacy experience and had no idea which I would prefer. Doing my first 6 months in (the) third year was good for me because I had such little pharmacy experience and ... it really helped me to learn when I returned to uni because I could relate back to my work experience. However, I also agree that doing the 5-year sandwich course does put lot of pressure on students in their final 6 months, especially in hospital, because there will always be that comparison between you and the 12-month students.'

TOP TIPS (FIFTH YEAR PLACEMENT)

- Make sure to remind everyone that you are a fifth year pre-reg on a sandwich programme
- If you have never been on a ward, remind everyone
- Remember that your pre-reg finishes in 6 months, not 12 months, as it does for others
- Remember that 6 months is not a long time and you are not squeezing 12 months of work into 6 months

---

TOP TIPS (THIRD YEAR PLACEMENT)

- Make sure to remind everyone that you are a third year pre-reg on a sandwich programme
- Keep your pre-reg portfolio from your first placement and bring this with you to your next placement
- Don't compare yourself with other pre-regs; you are not at the same stage as them
- Don't worry if you don't know the things that other pre-regs know
- Every experience is a good experience, so make the most of your experiences!

Primary care trusts

18

Pre-registration training placements in primary care trusts (PCTs) are a relatively new and expanding area. We feel that this area for pre-registration training is a growth area due to the increase in numbers of pharmacy graduates. In line with the industrial placements, PCT pre-reg placements must be split equally between a PCT and another sector – either community or hospital.

Although we recognise that this section applies to just a few hospitals, we also recognise that many hospitals may be looking to increase their pre-reg numbers or to expand the range of learning opportunities for their pre-regs. With this in mind we have decided to include this short section for those of you either considering hospital pre-reg programmes with a PCT rotation or joint hospital–PCT programmes, of which there is a growing number. This section should provide you with a brief insight into what it can be like having a rotation in a PCT.

PCT PHARMACY WORK

PCT pharmacy and medicines management teams vary greatly in terms of team structure and roles and responsibilities, and may encompass such work as working alongside other healthcare professionals to ensure that quality healthcare is delivered to the local population. There may also be some integration with social services, so therefore the boundaries may be blurred.

The core part of PCT pharmacy work is to analyse prescribing patterns of GP practices to ensure that GPs are working within national and local guidelines, and ensuring that healthcare professionals work within budgetary constraints. Pharmacy staff play a vital role in providing and analysing prescribing data to inform prescribers of their performance.

For a pre-reg, it may be a shock to discover that pharmacy work can be undertaken in an office environment! Although much of the work is done in the PCT offices, there are many opportunities for visiting surgeries and other healthcare professionals in their workplaces, so you will not be as tied to your desk as you might think.

THE ROLE OF THE PRE-REG WITHIN A PCT

Pre-regs play a large part in supporting many of the activities detailed below.

Analysing prescribing (ePact) data

This is an important job in that the data that are accessed via the NHS Business Services Authority (BSA) are analysed and fed back to the prescribers to compare their prescribing practices with national or local guidelines and with PCT or national averages. In this way, prescribers can review their prescribing practices to identify current good practice, plus areas where improvements can be made.

Prescribing reviews, including yearly updates on everything!

The pharmacy or medicines management department at the PCT is responsible for reviewing the prescribing patterns of their prescribers and updating prescribers on their budgetary standing. Using the ePact data analysis, pharmacy staff arrange review meetings with their GP practices to talk about their prescribing activities. In addition to this, pharmacists update the GPs on any new developments with drugs or with guidelines, to ensure that practice staff have relevant and up-to-date information. These updates are not just on clinical areas, but may also pertain to legal issues around drugs, e.g. safe and secure handling of drugs. This work exposes pre-regs to the legal aspects of drugs that may be examinable in the registration exam.

Clinic visits

You may be responsible for date checking stock, updating stock lists and writing reports to feed back results to clinic staff. Although this may seem like a technical activity, there are clinical elements involved here because you may be required to ascertain the clinical appropriateness of drugs on the clinic stock list.

GP practice audits

A pre-reg may be required to undertake audit work in a GP practice – the information gathered from the GP practice is audited against important national or local targets. This audit work can obviously be considered good evidence for the performance standard 'A4.8 Have successfully carried out a small, planned audit assignment'.

Training of healthcare professionals and patients, e.g. community inhaler counselling and cardiac rehab patients

As PCTs deliver locally responsive healthcare, this means that, for locally commissioned healthcare services, PCTs have to ensure that the healthcare professionals involved are well trained. Pharmacy is involved in these types of training, especially if the subject matter involves the use of drugs.

Providing pharmaceutical care to managed services: intermediate care, learning difficulties, etc.

This make take a similar form to that for your hospital colleagues, in that you may be required to undertake ward-like activities such as medicines reconciliation. Which clinical area this involves depends on the healthcare that the PCT provides in your local area.

Medicines information enquiry answering

Many clinical areas covered in medicines information (MI) involve answering enquiries. The difference in a PCT is that you may not have such a comprehensive library of resources that is available in a hospital MI centre.

Summarising national guidance such as NICE guidance and NPSA alerts

This may then progress into the production of 'flyers' which are distributed to PCT contractors such as GPs, community pharmacists, nursing staff.

Writing guidelines or documents relating to the safe and secure use of medicines

As part of a PCT's work, the medicines management and pharmacy departments are involved with producing many policies and procedures relating to medicines. There are many opportunities to be involved in this kind of work, which often involves attending meetings and collating people's opinions and comments.

Dissemination of national guidance for local use: cost comparisons of different pharmaceutical products using Drug Tariffs

When first discussing this placement with the Royal Pharmaceutical Society of Great Britain (RPSGB), we explored the ways in which the performance standards could be covered, because PCT pharmacy is not seen as mainstream pharmacy. Although it is correct that some of the performance standards cannot be covered, for example, it would be difficult to fulfil the dispensing and checking requirements (performance standards: 'C1 Manage the dispensing process') if you are not based in a dispensary environment, it can also be said that the work that a pre-reg undertakes WILL cover most of the performance standards because many of these cover how pre-regs manage themselves, their work, their learning and their interpersonal skills.

As can be seen from the above examples, many of the pieces of work with which a pre-reg can get involved require working with a wide variety of healthcare professionals and communicating in a number of ways (performance standards 'B1 Communicate effectively' and 'B2 Work effectively with others'), working to an agreed high standard. Also, a lot of your day-to-day work may involve answering MI enquiries for GP practice staff and clinic staff on a wide range of clinical areas (performance standards 'C2 Provide additional clinical and pharmaceutical services').

Some pre-regs will be concerned with the lack of 'clinical' work. We would dispute this, because we feel that pharmacy in all sectors is 'clinical'. Although there may be little day-to-day contact, there can be no dispute that pre-regs will be working with the latest up-to-date national and local guidance and asked to interpret the clinical and pharmaceutical aspects contained within. In the PCT, pre-regs also learn about how differently pharmacy can influence prescribing. They may well be involved with influencing many clinical practitioners by producing flyers or newsletters proactively providing them with information. This differs greatly to practice in other sectors; in hospital or community pharmacy, at pre-reg stage, your influence is as one pre-reg to one clinical practitioner, or one patient, whereas, at the PCT, by undertaking one piece of work, one pre-reg can influence ALL the clinical practitioners in that PCT.

Although hospital timetables involve rotations through different areas, requiring you just to turn up to the right place at the right time, you will have the additional responsibility of organising your own time and your own workload, because no one else will do this for you. This will give you extra evidence for hitting the 'A1 Managing self' performance standard.

In addition, added benefits come from working in a smaller team, because your role as a pre-reg may involve extra responsibilities to which your community or hospital counterparts may not be exposed. A major component to this is the additional responsibility that you may have to take for your own learning. Experiences at a PCT will definitely propel you into thinking and acting like a pharmacist.

'At first I didn't know what to expect from my PCT placement. I got given work on the first day, work that got given to GPs. I saw that my presence was having an impact straight away. I started off on enquiry answering which was the same as answering enquiries in MI and so this did not feel strange. A couple of months in, I was working jointly with the pharmacists. Then I did a statin audit in GP practices and went in on my own to identify patients eligible to be switched onto different statins. I had a lot of responsibility, but the end decision was still with the GP. It was great that I had real input and that what I was saying was actually listened to.'

'The work at the PCT has been linking well with the performance standards. For instance I worked on the new antihypertensive guidelines and it highlighted to me that I actually know quite a lot. I definitely achieved tasks and was in situations where I was hitting performance standards without even realising it. I was definitely achieving performance standards through-out the placement.'

'I think that I think quite differently now, I'm not so narrow focused. Probably for 3 days a week I'm doing the same as the other pre-regs but coming at if from a different viewpoint, that's all.'

'I went from very structured rotations to no structure at the PCT, which has made me think about my own work and how to organise myself; I have to recognise what my own workload is and actively find things to do to plug gaps in my own knowledge. I used to be spoon fed, but the PCT is totally different; I am organising myself here.'

'I think that I have changed a lot. I feel that I have the power to sort myself out. I have that control now. It was difficult at first but now I take more responsibility for my own development. I am becoming more confident about what I know and don't know.'

'I thoroughly enjoyed the PCT – if I were to do my pre-reg again, I would still do the PCT placement. It has made me think so differently from the other pre-regs. Although there was little direct patient contact I have learnt lots of different things.'

TOP TIPS

- PCT work is challenging in its own way
- Be prepared for extra responsibility for your own development when in the PCT
- Be prepared to learn a lot about local and national NHS initiatives
- Think about the patient at population rather than individual level

Pharmaceutical industry 19

There are very few industrial placements compared with the number of placements for community and hospital pharmacy. There is sometimes a misconception that industrial placements suit only the geeky scientist because the work mainly relates to the science of formulation and requires you to be very pharmaceutically minded. The reality is very different because no industrial placement is without a patient facing hospital or community experience, which is needed to meet the requirements of the performance standards programme. You will be surprised how many transferable skills you gain from working in the industrial sector. Sometimes you may think that by doing an industrial placement you do not need to see or speak to patients, or people, and that you are happier working in laboratories doing your own projects. Nothing could be further from the truth because, even if you are not talking to patients, you will definitely be talking to people, and negotiating and influencing them to get what you need for your project. You may even come into conflict with people and need to learn how to manage these situations.

Most industrial placements involve 6 months in each sector although, for some placements, there can be little communication between the two sets of pre-reg tutors, or what communication there is can be based on incorrect assumptions about each sector in terms of what is required by the pre-reg and how the standards are signed off during each placement. It is up to you to ensure that you are aware of what is required of you in both placements and that you have a good understanding of the performance standards, so that you can guide your supervisors or tutor re. what to sign off and what can be assessed in the next placement.

The first 6 months in a hospital is generally the same as for the other pre-regs, except that you have less time to complete all that you need to do; either you have fewer rotations than the 12-month pre-regs or you spend less time in the rotations. The difficulty is that, because you will not be in direct patient contact for the industrial placement, you have to ensure that you have made the most of every learning opportunity presented to you and that you have gathered enough evidence to satisfy your tutor that you are competent in the performance standards for which it is difficult to claim in the industrial placement. This means that you have to settle in a bit quicker than the other pre-regs and perhaps work a bit harder earlier on because you have less time. It also means that you need to develop organisational and time management skills, particularly if these are not your forte.

An example of this can be seen from this comment in the box.

> 'I'm worried that I don't have enough time to get my dispensing right, I have no experience of community pharmacy and I can't dispense at the moment. I keep making lots of dispensing errors and they are not the same thing all the time. . . . I think I may need more time in the dispensary.'

One of the worries that you may have is that you may be disadvantaged by doing your industrial placement second and, in the build-up to the registration exam, you are not in a mainstream placement. This is not a problem because the pass rate for the industrial placement pre-regs is no different to any other pre-reg and the pre-reg tutors in the industrial placements provide lots of support. Also, it is always a good idea to stay in contact with the hospital pre-regs and the hospital pre-reg tutor, if you can, so that they can help you with any worries or concerns that you may have in the build-up to the exam.

One of our pre-regs made the comment in the box, highlighting a common misconception and concern.

> 'I'm not sure if I will be able to revise for the exam properly because I'll be stuck in a lab all day and won't have access to people whom I can ask questions. The people in [the industry] won't be practising pharmacists and won't know how to answer my questions.'

The problem that you might have is adapting very quickly to the industrial sector and the different ways of working when you change after 6 months – after all you are going from a hospital environment, where a lot of your time has been spent dealing with patient-related problems and the people working with you are all from pharmacy. In the industrial sector, you work with non-pharmacists as well as pharmacists.

Coming to the hospital for your second placement can be more difficult because you will have spent your first 6 months in industry working with possibly fewer pre-regs and definitely fewer pharmacists, and concentrated on one main project that was pharmaceutical in nature. You will come to the hospital placement with skills developed in working by yourself, prioritising and managing your own time, as well as negotiating with others to be able to complete your project. You will probably find the life of a hospital pre-reg very different and will, in some respects, be in a similar position to pre-regs who are starting their training year. The only difference is that you have much less time to settle in and acclimatise to the work that you have to do. Although you have an induction to hospital pharmacy, you will find that you may have to join an existing team of pre-regs and, in that respect, you are no different to the Bradford sandwich course pre-regs. The fundamental difference for you is that you do not have a whole 6 months because the last month does not really count with the registration exam coming at the end of July. Taking out the induction and settling-in period, you probably only have 4 of the 6 months to complete the work that you need to do, prepare for the registration exam and prepare for being a qualified pharmacist at the end of the 6 months. This is a massive challenge and one to which you should be able to rise!

One of the main challenges that you encounter is the fact that you are in the second half of your training and seen as such by the staff around you. They probably expect you to be able to work at the same level as the pre-regs in the 12-month programme. You can't do this at the start but should be able to do it by the end of your training. You pre-reg tutor is instrumental in guiding you through your placement so it is critical that you meet him or her early, set out your goals and define the standards for working. It is very important to be honest to yourself and discuss your own strengths, weaknesses and experience of mainstream pharmacy so that your training can be tailored to suit your needs. You also need to be careful that you do not benchmark your practice against that of the other pre-regs and do not feel that you are in any way lower or less knowledgeable than them – you are doing a different training programme and cannot be expected to know as much as they do. After all, how much pharmaceutical and formulation science have the others been exposed to?

You think about problems differently to the other pre-regs because you see things as they are and won't necessarily be used to the workplace culture of the area where you are working. You may even question why that particular task needs to be done in that particular area or on that particular workbench. Be careful to talk to the other pre-regs, and perhaps even your tutor, to find out who is who in the area in which you are working.

As a scientist in the purest sense, sometimes industrial pre-regs think in a black-and-white way, i.e. there is only one correct answer; you will quickly realise that real-life practice is just not like that. There are no textbook patients with just one problem; they often have more than one co-morbidity or they would not be in hospital.

The industrial placement is a unique placement in many senses because you work in completely different sectors, but have the advantage of learning so many transferable skills that you come out of the pre-registration time completely different to a traditional pre-reg. The exam stress can be unfounded because you are in the same boat as the others and you build up to the exam with the others, so have an opportunity to learn from them and they from you.

In terms of career opportunities, although it may be true that many industrial pre-regs go on to do PhDs and work in the pharmaceutical industry, there are many others who never return to industry and make their careers in hospital or community pharmacy. At the end of the day, the career choice is up to you and no one puts any pressure on you to pursue a particular career – just that, with an industrial placement under your belt, different opportunities are open to you.

TOP TIPS

- Pharmaceutical industry is not just for scientists
- In the pharmaceutical industry you are at the 'other end' of patient care in terms of drug discovery and drug design
- You learn lots of transferable skills in an industrial placement
- Make the most of the hospital experience because it provides you with a valuable insight into how patients manage their medicines
- The registration exam is important, but not as important as your pre-reg experience

---

Specialist focus: paediatrics 20

We have included this short section to provide an example of specialist rotations because many hospitals have rotations that are in specialist areas. From our experience, these can be in such specialist clinical areas as oncology and haematology, and in specialist hospitals such as heart and lung and children's hospitals. We have decided to include this short section to highlight that there are many transferable skills and lots of knowledge can be gained from working in a specialist rotation for transfer into your mainstream practice. Paediatrics is just an example that we have chosen to show that it can be a generalist area within a specialism (if you get what we mean!).

Saying that paediatrics is a specialist area is like saying that 'adults' is one too! That simply doesn't make sense. Just as there are many things that can go wrong for adults resulting in many different branches of adult medicine, so it is with paediatric medicine.

'Paediatrics was very different, a completely different world. Things that are not important in adults are very important in children. I spent most of afternoons looking things up!'

There is a lot more to paediatrics than just simply considering children as smaller versions of adults. At different times in a child's life, there are different processes and developments happening, which means that, at different stages of children's lives, children handle drugs differently so it is not just a case of seeing them as 'little people'. The dosing of medicines in paediatrics tends to be very closely based on weight or body surface area. It can be a challenge keeping track of the correct dosage for a child because a child's weight can change quickly. Another issue is that many medicines routinely used in adult medicine are not licensed for use in children, even when the drug is used in common practice.

'Working with unlicensed medicines is difficult. If I'm happy and it's common knowledge then that's fine.'

The types of children whom you may see may depend on how big the paediatric department is. Most district general hospitals have one or two general paediatric wards. These wards house any children who may have been admitted for a number of different reasons. Many of the patients whom you encounter were previously fit and well children who may have come into hospital after banging their head, or suffering from an infection, fit or an episode of difficulty in breathing. For many of these cases, admission into hospital is for precautionary measures and monitoring, and most make a full recovery. For a small proportion of these children, a subsequent diagnosis of some long-term condition may be made that necessitates referral to a specialist paediatric centre. You may also see another type of child – one who is already under the care of a specialist centre, but the main bulk of care takes place in the local hospital because of convenience and travel purposes. In these cases, the medical notes of the patients have detailed treatment plans that should not be deviated from without prior knowledge of the specialist centre administering the main care.

'I didn't like paediatrics. All you do are drug histories; all everybody is on is paracetamol, and ibuprofen and that's it. Just come from Gen Med where I had quite a lot of responsibility. It seemed always to be the same drugs, and then just a few patients who were complicated.'

If you work in a specialist paediatric hospital, then, just as with adult medicine, there are cardiac wards, surgical wards, neurology wards, high-dependency units, etc., as well as wards for general paediatric admissions. In this setting, you will obviously see a wider range of paediatric specialities, with the prospect of seeing more complicated cases.

CALCULATIONS, CALCULATIONS, CALCULATIONS!

In paediatrics, you would expect to calculate, check and recheck each and every dose. Although for adult medicine, many medicines are a fixed dose, in paediatrics the dose changes with the weight of the child. Also the milligram per kilogram dose of medicines may change in the lifetime of a child because children of different ages handle drugs differently, depending on how developed their organ functions are. For injectable drugs, to ensure that the correct dilution has been made, you also need to work out displacement values, rates and concentrations. All these calculations are useful in preparation for your exams. One advantage of doing calculations on a daily basis is that it takes the fear away from doing them, because you become used to doing them.

DEALING WITH VERY SICK YOUNG CHILDREN: THE EMOTIONS

Dealing with children and babies who may be very sick is usually emotionally very difficult. If you love children it may be difficult to see them in distress or pain. It can be even more distressing when the parents or family accepts the situation! Try to be professional and think of how you can help as opposed to dwelling on the fact that you may be presented with a child who may not have much of a future in your eyes. When a child dies it can be quite a shock. Although you could expect older people to die, the shock of a child dying may be greater, especially if it is an unexpected death.

'I was very apprehensive about the paediatric rotation. I didn't think I was emotionally strong enough to deal with sick children. Some days are better than others. Some days it breaks my heart. It makes you look at your life and not be sorry and not complain. On a pharmacist level, not doing anything is not an option. I have to make sure I do things right. I didn't know how important age and weights are until now.'

DEALING WITH THE PARENTS RATHER THAN THE CHILDREN THEMSELVES

As many of the children are too young to speak to healthcare professionals, your primary contact may be with the child's parents or carers. Although many parents are knowledgeable about their child's condition and have the child's welfare and wellbeing at heart, some parents aren't, and that may also be hard to take. Remember that parents may have a set of health beliefs that opposes those of recognised western medicine, and they may refuse treatment on behalf of their child if the treatment opposes their own views.

'Many of the children are so young they cannot talk. One 13-year-old patient I saw had a spinal injury. I mainly interacted with the father, as the patient was unable to give any information as they were in so much pain. Obviously if you ask a relative information you need to question if the information is truthful, so you need to be careful of information sources and information given.'

'On the general paediatric ward I took a lot of drug histories and dispensed a lot of TTOs. For the drug histories you have to rely on the patients' carers. I saw lots of different disease states – asthma, TB, sickle cell, constipation. There are definitely differences between adults and children. For children the drug history taking is slightly different and lots of children did not swallow tablets.'

'Before paediatrics, I didn't know what form any drug came in, but here formulation is so important.'

MANY COMMON SKILLS NO MATTER WHAT CLINICAL AREA

Although you may have trained in a 'specialist' area such as paediatrics, this does not mean that you have limited yourself. Just as with adult medicine, the clinical area that you are in does not really matter, because you are learning some generic ward-based skills around problem-solving, dealing with other healthcare professionals, prioritising your workload, etc. Much of the pre-reg training year is about getting you do learn how to do things, and whether you have spent a lot of time in elderly care, orthopaedics or paediatrics, the aims of providing pharmaceutical care are always to ensure that the patient comes to no harm. Many of the problem-solving, multidisciplinary working and communication skills that you exercise in paediatrics are widely applicable to a multitude of other situations involving other patient groups.

Be mindful, however, that a large part of the registration exam at the end of your pre-reg year focuses on common ADULT medicines, because much of the paediatric care that you may provide is too specialised. If you do not come into contact with adult medicine during your year, make sure that you familiarise yourself with the common medicines that adults take for common conditions such as hypertension and myocardial infarction, asthma and chronic obstructive pulmonary disease (COPD), pain control and infectious diseases. If you do not see any adult patients in a hospital setting, it would be wise to concentrate on the adult prescriptions that you may see on your community cross-sector experience, because, with these prescriptions, you are likely to encounter the common drugs that many adults are being treated with.

TOP TIPS

- Children are not little adults
- Doses matter and can be larger than those for adults on a milligram per kilogram basis
- Calculations are critical
- The formulation and routes of medicines matter
- Small children in hospital are the same small children in community
- Speaking with parents and carers is different to speaking to patients
- Some young children can be experts in their own medicines

Section 7

Future issues

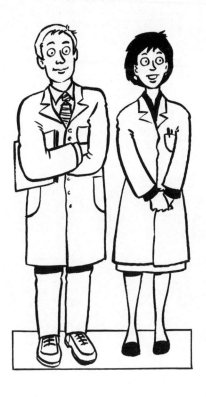

The future: gazing at the crystal ball

21

We hope that we have taken you through the journey of what is probably the most pivotal and fundamental year of your career. This is the year where you start out as a student fresh from university and, hopefully, end as a fully qualified pharmacist. At the end of every training year we always ask our pre-regs to remember what is was like for them at the start of their pre-reg year and to keep that memory when training the pharmacists of the future, because these pre-regs will come to you with the same issues and problems.

As always with healthcare and the NHS there are many changes taking place in the wider healthcare environment, in the pharmacy profession itself and, more importantly for you, in pharmacy education. The changes in pharmacy education that may affect you relate to integrating the undergraduate degree with practice and focusing more on the clinical aspects of being a pharmacist; remember, however, what we thought when we described 'clinical' practice.

Proposed future changes will mean that there may not be a pre-reg year or pre-reg placements as they currently exist. There may be more frequent, shorter placements throughout your degree programme, which could mean receiving the training, assessment and feedback at the level of a pharmacist (whatever that is) rather than at the level of an undergraduate student (whatever that is). We anticipate that these changes will take some years to come into effect and that there will be some changes to pharmacy practice, e.g. dealing with more advanced, novel and innovative therapies such as biomedicines, where the knowledge base is different but progression is always there in terms of developing healthcare. There may be more pharmacists prescribing, greater links with primary care and, hopefully, a break down of the existing care sectors so that all healthcare is integrated and community, hospital and primary care pharmacists all work together with a common goal.

Prevention of diseases and conditions needs pharmacists at the coalface with the appropriate skills and knowledge to act as gatekeepers for our patients and to refer them to the right person. Not to say that we don't do this already, just that, as all our school reports used to say, 'we could do better'!

The main thing to say at the end of this book is that the future of pharmacy does not really depend on us, who have written this book and are practising at the moment, but on YOU. It is you who will be training future undergraduates and future pharmacists and it is you who will be developing the profession and, again hopefully, 'going where no man has gone before' in terms of progressing the role of the pharmacist in caring for our patients and the general public. Don't be scared to embrace the future and make a real difference.

Lastly, we end with the quote that we started this book with, in the hope that it makes more sense now:

'A wise man learns from experience; an even wiser man learns from the experience of others…' Plato (424–423 BC to 348–347 BC).

Now go and make the future of pharmacy!

Index

spectators, team, 22
staff, dispensary, 62
standard operating procedures (SOPs)
  community pharmacy, 90, 92
  dispensary, 62
  technical services, 78, 79, 80
sterile products, manufacture, 78
stock checks, 61
stores, 66
students
  community pharmacy placements,
    85, 87
  other, 16
  sandwich courses *see* sandwich
    courses, integrated
  transition to work, 4, 37, 38, 39, 40
study days, regional, 17, 88
substance misuse, 99
supervision, 53, 55
supervisors, 45
  assessment by, 104
  end-of-rotation reviews, 112
syllabus, registration exam, 133

tablets, identifying, 73
tea breaks, 62, 88
team(s)
  dynamics, 23
  getting to know your, 15–16, 19
  qualities of bad, 22
  qualities of good, 21
  roles, 25
  working in, 19
technical services, 77
  assessment in, 109, 110
terminally ill children, 169
terrorists, team, 23

timekeeping, 6
total parenteral nutrition (TPN), 77, 80
Tuckman's model of groups, 23
tutors, 12, 14, 31
  getting to know, 31
  industrial placements, 163
  managing your, 33
  potential problems, 35
  RPSGB progress reviews, 40, 112
  sandwich course placements, 150
  signing off by, 111
  working with, 47

United Kingdom Medicines Information
    (UKMI) workbook, 70, 109
unlicensed medicines
  paediatrics, 167
  preparation, 78
  quality assurance, 83

vials, 81

wards
  assessment on, 106, 107
  rotations, 49, 153
  stock top-ups, 66
websites, advertising jobs, 122
work
  making transition to, 4, 37, 38, 39, 40
  as a professional pharmacist, 41, 121
  see also job
working hours, 123
workplace
  getting to know, 11, 12, 15
  induction period, 14
written correspondence, 74